LYMPHOPROLIFERATIVE DISEASES:
PATHOGENESIS, DIAGNOSIS, THERAPY

DEVELOPMENTS IN ONCOLOGY

F.J. Cleton and J.W.I.M. Simons, eds., Genetic Origins of Tumour Cells. ISBN 90-247-2272-1
J. Aisner and P. Chang, eds., Cancer Treatment Research. ISBN 90-247-2358-2
B.W. Ongerboer de Visser, D.A. Bosch and W.M.H. van Woerkom-Eykenboom, eds., Neuro-oncology: Clinical and Experimental Aspects. ISBN 90-247-2421-X
K. Hellmann, P. Hilgard and S. Eccles, eds., Metastasis: Clinical and Experimental Aspects. ISBN 90-247-2424-4
H.F. Seigler, ed., Clinical Management of Melanoma. ISBN 90-247-2584-4
P. Correa and W. Haenszel, eds., Epidemiology of Cancer of the Digestive Tract. ISBN 90-247-2601-8
L.A. Liotta and I.R. Hart, eds., Tumour Invasion and Metastasis. ISBN 90-247-2611-5
J. Bánóczy, ed., Oral Leukoplakia. ISBN 90-247-2655-7
C. Tijssen, M. Halprin and L. Endtz, eds., Familial Brain Tumours. ISBN 90-247-2691-3
F.M. Muggia, C.W. Young and S.K. Carter, eds., Anthracycline Antibiotics in Cancer. ISBN 90-247-2711-1
B.W. Hancock, ed., Assessment of Tumour Response. ISBN 90-247-2712-X
D.E. Peterson, ed., Oral Complications of Cancer Chemotherapy. ISBN 0-89838-563-6
R. Mastrangelo, D.G. Poplack and R. Riccardi, eds., Central Nervous System Leukemia. Prevention and Treatment. ISBN 0-89838-570-9
A. Polliack, ed., Human Leukemias. Cytochemical and Ultrastructural Techniques in Diagnosis and Research. ISBN 0-89838-585-7
W. Davis, C. Maltoni and S. Tanneberger, eds., The Control of Tumor Growth and its Biological Bases. ISBN 0-89838-603-9
A.P.M. Heintz, C.Th. Griffiths and J.B. Trimbos, eds., Surgery in Gynecological Oncology. ISBN 0-89838-604-7
M.P. Hacker, E.B. Double and I. Krakoff, eds., Platinum Coordination Complexes in Cancer Chemotherapy. ISBN 0-89838-619-5
M.J. van Zwieten, The Rat as Animal Model in Breast Cancer Research: A Histopathological Study of Radiation- and Hormone-Induced Rat Mammary Tumors. ISBN 0-89838-624-1
B. Löwenberg and A. Hagenbeek, eds., Minimal Residual Disease in Acute Leukemia. ISBN 0-89838-630-6
I. van der Waal and G.B. Snow, eds., Oral Oncology. ISBN 0-89838-631-4
B.W. Hancock and A.H. Ward, eds., Immunological Aspects of Cancer. ISBN 0-89838-664-0
K.V. Honn and B.F. Sloane, Hemostatic Mechanisms and Metastasis. ISBN 0-89838-667-5
K.R. Harrap, W. Davis and A.H. Calvert, eds., Cancer Chemotherapy and Selective Drug Development. ISBN 0-89838-673-X
C.J.H. van de Velde and P.H. Sugarbaker, eds., Liver Metastasis. ISBN 0-89838-648-5
D.J. Ruiter, K. Welvaart and S. Ferrone, eds., Cutaneous Melanoma and Precursor Lesions. ISBN 0-89838-689-6
S.B. Howell, ed., Intra-arterial and Intracavitary Cancer Chemotherapy. ISBN 0-89838-691-8
D.L. Kisner and J.F. Smyth, eds., Interferon Alpha-2: Pre-Clinical and Clinical Evaluation. ISBN 0-89838-701-9
P. Furmanski, J.C. Hager and M.A. Rich, eds., RNA Tumor Viruses, Oncogenes, Human Cancer and Aids: On the Frontiers of Understanding. ISBN 0-89838-703-5
J. Talmadge, I.J. Fidler and R.K. Oldham, Screening for Biological Response Modifiers: Methods and Rationale. ISBN 0-89838-712-4
J.C. Bottino, R.W. Opfell and F.M. Muggia, eds., Liver Cancer. ISBN 0-89838-713-2
P.K. Pattengale, R.J. Lukes and C.R. Taylor, Lymphoproliferative diseases: pathogenesis, diagnosis, therapy. ISBN 0-89838-725-6

LYMPHOPROLIFERATIVE DISEASES: PATHOGENESIS, DIAGNOSIS, THERAPY

Proceedings of a symposium presented at the University of Southern California, Department of Pathology and the Kenneth J. Norris Cancer Hospital and Research Institute, Los Angeles, U.S.A., November 16–17, 1984

edited by

Paul K. Pattengale, M.D.
Robert J. Lukes, M.D.
Clive R. Taylor, M.B., B.Chir., D.Phil.
Hematopathology Section, Department of Pathology
U.S.C. School of Medicine, Los Angeles, California

1985 **MARTINUS NIJHOFF PUBLISHERS**
a member of the KLUWER ACADEMIC PUBLISHERS GROUP
BOSTON / DORDRECHT / LANCASTER

Distributors

for the United States and Canada: Kluwer Academic Publishers, 190 Old Derby Street, Hingham, MA 02043, USA
for the UK and Ireland: Kluwer Academic Publishers, MTP Press Limited, Falcon House, Queen Square, Lancaster LA1 1RN, UK
for all other countries: Kluwer Academic Publishers Group, Distribution Center, P.O. Box 322, 3300 AH Dordrecht, The Netherlands

Library of Congress Cataloging in Publication Data

Library of Congress Cataloging in Publication Data
Main entry under title:

Lymphoproliferative diseases.

(Developments in oncology)
Includes index.
1. Lymphoproliferative disorders--Congresses.
I. Pattengale, Paul K. II. Lukes, Robert J.
III. Taylor, C. R. (Clive Roy) IV. University of Southern California. Dept. of Pathology. V. Kenneth J. Norris Cancer Hospital and Research Institute.
RC646.2.L96 1985 616.99'442 85-5071

ISBN-13: 978-94-010-8721-6 e-ISBN-13: 978-94-009-5016-0
DOI: 10.1007/978-94-009-5016-0

TABLE OF CONTENTS

DIAGNOSIS

CLINICAL ASPECTS

Symposium Faculty

Gunther Dennert, Ph.D.
USC-Department of Microbiology
2025 Zonal Avenue
Los Angeles, CA 90033

Kenneth Foon, M.D.
Clinical Investigation Section
NCI, NIH, Medical Pavilion
335 Park Avenue
Frederick, MD 21701

Warner Greene, M.D.
Metabolism Branch
NIH, Bldg. 10, Rm. 4N-117
Bethesda, MD 20205

Samuel Halpern, M.D.
Department of Radiology
Veterans' Administration Hospital
3350 La Jolla Village Drive
San Diego, CA 92161

Hans Hansen, Ph.D.
Director of Research
Ortho Diagnostic Systems, Inc.
Raritan, NJ 08869

George Klein, M.D.
Department of Tumor Biology
Institut for Tumorbiologi
Karolinska Institutet, Box 60400
104 01 Stockholm, Sweden

Stanley Korsmeyer, M.D.
Metabolism Branch
NIH, Bldg. 10, Rm. 4N-107
Bethesda, MD 20205

Alexandra Levine, M.D.
USC-Division of Hematology
2025 Zonal Avenue
Los Angeles, CA 90033

Robert Lukes, M.D.
USC-Department of Pathology
2025 Zonal Avenue
Los Angeles, CA 90033

Paul Meyer, M.D.
USC-Department of Pathology
2025 Zonal Avenue
Los Angeles, CA 90033

John Parker, M.D.
USC-Department of Pathology
2025 Zonal Avenue
Los Angeles, CA 90033

Paul Pattengale, M.D.
USC-Department of Pathology
2025 Zonal Avenue
Los Angeles, CA 90033

Saul Rosenberg, M.D.
Division of Oncology
Stanford University
Stanford, CA 94035

Ronald Ross, M.D.
USC-Department of
Preventive Medicine
2025 Zonal Avenue
Los Angeles, CA 90033

Kazuo Tajima, M.D.
Aichi Cancer Center
Chikusa-Ku
Nagoya, Japan

Clive R. Taylor, M.D., D.Phil.
USC-Department of Pathology
2025 Zonal Avenue
Los Angeles, CA 90033

Dedicated to

ROBERT J. LUKES, M.D.

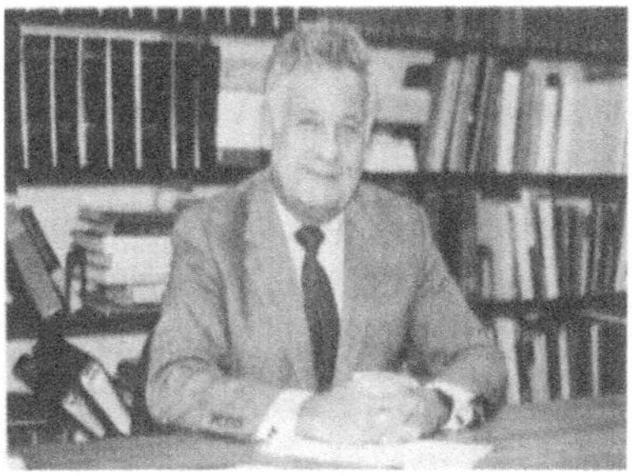

on the occasion of his retirement from the Los Angeles County/ University of Southern California Medical Center for his years of dedicated service to the diagnosis of lymphoproliferative diseases.

Dr. Robert J. Lukes has made a major impact on the field of hematopathology. His contributions to the diagnosis and understanding of Hodgkin's disease and lymphomas have been numerous and seminal. He began his published contributions with an important description of Korean epidemic hemorrhagic fever while stationed in Korea in 1951-1953. It was in this paper that he began to demonstrate his ability to correlate pathologic, physiologic and clinical manifestations of disease and their relationship to the evolution of that disease. This set the tone for his future investigations and publications as he refined the approach so that it became a hallmark of his writings and teaching. His colleagues have always been impressed by his astounding ability to examine histologic material from numbers of cases of poorly understood or undefined disease entities, select unifying features, correlate them and develop a hypothesis for the pathogenesis of the entity. He developed this ability during his tenure at the Armed Forces Institute of Pathology between 1953 and 1962 where he had the opportunity to examine several thousand cases of Hodgkin's disease and non-Hodgkin's lymphomas and leukemias. He recognized early in this experience that if he applied an analytical approach to explaining each feature of the histology in these diseases and attempted to relate the histological findings to the physiological and clinical findings the histologic case material would be his greatest teacher.

His initial study of Hodgkin's disease was one involving 377 cases, in collaboration with Dr. James Butler. This led to a description of the pathology of Hodgkin's disease in a new and exciting way and resulted in six new distinctive histologic types which were related to clinical stages and to survival. One of the most important outcomes of this study was the identification of a type of Hodgkin's disease, nodular sclerosis, which had been previously unrecognized. This particular type proved to be unique, since survival was better than with other types, and it appeared to be different than the other histologic types in evolution. Following this initial description, Dr. Lukes chaired a committee on the morphology of Hodgkin's disease at the Rye Conference in 1966. Under his leadership, the group proposed a classification of Hodgkin's disease which included four major types. These could be associated with clinical behavior, and this "Rye Classification" has stood the test of time. Its value and international acceptance have been apparent to workers in the field as evidenced by the fact that it is used in essentially all studies where pathologic classification is required. This new classification, in conjunction with newly developed clinical staging categories, completely changed the outlook for patients with Hodgkin's disease. It provided prognostically useful histologic features which are of aid in determining therapy. Along with his colleagues in pathology and radiology, Dr. Lukes, by correlating histological type, clinical features and response to therapy, clearly demonstrated the clinical value of his classification and helped eliminate any doubt that Hodgkin's disease can be cured if appropriately treated. In subsequent years Dr. Lukes and colleagues helped clarify the nature of the Reed-Sternberg cell, its diagnostic usefulness and the role of Reed-Sternberg cells and variants in the process of Hodgkin's disease.

Not satisfied with the major contributions he made to the diagnosis and understanding of Hodgkin's disease, and after joining the faculty at the University of Southern California School of Medicine in 1962, Dr. Lukes began to concentrate on the non-Hodgkin's lymphomas. Initial investigations of the lymphocyte transformation phenomenon with Dr. John W. Parker starting in 1964 demonstrated that the morphological changes which occurred when small lymphocytes transform into dividing blast cells provide an in vitro model for events that occur in response to antigens in lymphoid tissues in vivo. It was this phenomenon that ultimately led to his proposal that lymphomas are the result of a block or "switch on" of the lymphocyte transformation mechanism.

In the late 1960's, utilizing the information obtained from these lymphocyte transformation studies and correlating this with the histological features of the many lymphomas he was seeing, Dr. Lukes began to develop a "functional approach for malignant lymphomas." This ultimately led to the Lukes/Collins classification. Once again he utilized his unique ability to convert static images of stained histologic sections into a dynamic view of the spectrum of events occurring in vivo. In his eyes, many isolated "still" pictures of histologic material are seen as frames in a developing movie.

The Lukes/Collins classification that arose from this approach was based on the idea that B cell lymphomas arising in the follicles of lymphoid tissue represent arrests in the normal transformation of lymphocytes. Similarly T cell lymphomas arise in the paracortex. Lukes predicted that because of their location and cytological characteristics, lymphomas could be classified as T or B lymphocytic in origin even without any confirming immunological markers. This prediction was soon confirmed by applying immunological markers to lymphoma phenotyping. As an outcome of this "functional approach to the diagnosis of lymphomas," it is now common-place to refer to lymphomas and leukemias of different cell types as frozen stages in ontogeny. It has also become clear that certain entities which can be distinguished histologically and phenotyped as B or T cell proliferations have different prognoses and will respond to therapy differently. An excellent example is found in the immunoblastic sarcomas of B and T cell type in which prognosis and behavior differ between the two.

Several new morphological and clinical entities have developed from utilization of this new classification. The classification has already identified homogeneous groups for comparison of treatment modalities and for determining prognosis and survival much more precise than those provided by previous classifications. It is predictable that the results of his studies of the non-Hodgkin's lymphomas will have an even greater ultimate impact than those achieved in Hodgkin's disease.

His colleagues who have worked with him closely over the years have never ceased to be amazed at Dr. Lukes' uncanny ability to recognize, analyze and synthesize information from histologic material. His ability to stimulate the thinking and investigations of his colleagues, not only those who work with him but those who hear his frequent lectures throughout the world, is clearly apparent from the many publications which either refer to his work or are the direct result of his observations and hypotheses. Probably most affected by his teaching are the numerous visiting fellows from the United States and other countries who have spent time with him, studying the variety of unusual lymphomas, leukemias and Hodgkin's disease that come across his desk daily. His ability to stimulate their imagination, excite them with his ideas, involve them in investigative projects and treat them in the kind and gentlemanly fashion that is his nature has had a major impact on their careers.

Because of the many important contributions to the field of Hodgkin's disease and the lymphoproliferative disorders, this symposium has been given in his honor and this book is dedicated to him.

John W. Parker, M.D.
University of Southern California

ONCOGENE ACTIVATION BY CHROMOSOMAL TRANSLOCATIONS

GEORGE KLEIN

The purpose of this paper is to document and discuss in detail some recent studies on chromosome translocations (reviewed in reference 1) which tie together the fields of cytogenetics and oncogene research (reviewed in reference 2).

In studying the cytogenetics of various tumors, it was discovered in two entirely different systems--one in a mouse B cell tumor (plasmacytoma) and the other in a human B cell tumor (Burkitt's lymphoma) that there were convergent chromosomal findings. Firstly, mouse plasmacytomas demonstrate two important cytogenetic changes, as seen in Figure 1. The most frequent one, which is called a typical change, involves the translocation of a portion of chromosome 15 to the distal portion of chromosome 12. The more infrequent or variant translocation also involves the same distal band of chromosome 15, which now translocates to chromosome 6. When this was observed, it was already known that chromosome 12 carried the immunoglobulin heavy chain (IgH) locus and that chromosome 6 carried the kappa light chain locus. It was also known that B cell tumors with this 15/6 translocation were kappa producers. It was therefore hypothesized that, since these were immunoglobulin-producing tumors, perhaps there was an oncogene located somewhere on the distal part of chromosome 15, which had somehow come under the influence of a transcriptionally active, chromosomal immunoglobulin (Ig) gene region, leading to activation of the oncogene, and thus resulting in a B cell tumor. The findings of Hayward et al[3] that, in avian B cell lymphomas, the insertion of a retrovirus next to the cellular oncogene c-myc led to the activation of that oncogene, also influenced this hypothesis. In the case of plasmacytomas, it was hypothesized that it would not be a virus activation mechanism, but rather a cellular activation mechanism. Although at first rather tentative, the hypothesis proved to be correct, since an oncogene was localized right at the

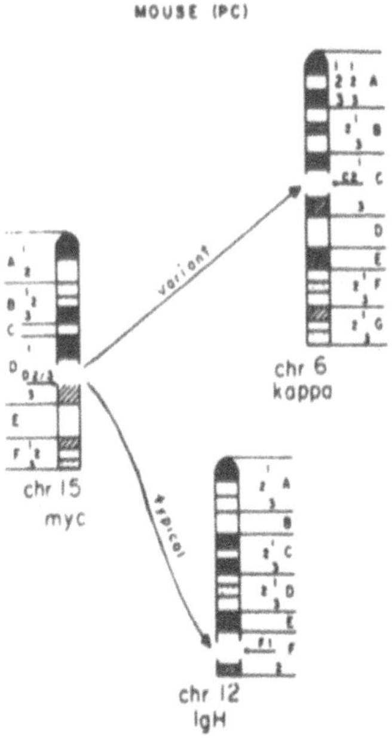

FIGURE 1. Schematic representation of typical and variant translocations involving c-myc on chromosome 15 in mouse plasmacytomas (PC). The typical translocation (15/12) involves the movement of c-myc to the immunoglobulin heavy chain locus (IgH) on chromosome 12. The variant translocation (15/6) involves the movement of c-myc to the kappa light chain locus on chromosome 6.

---

breakpoint on chormosome 15. It proved to be c-myc, the same oncogene which was found by Hayward et al[3] in the promotor insertion model of bursa-derived B cell chicken lymphoma.

The hypothesis actually became more plausible long before the myc oncogene was discovered, since a similar set of cytogenetic findings were made on Burkitt's lymphoma cells. In B cell-derived Burkitt's lymphoma, it was first observed that there was a characteristic marker called 14q+, which was characterized by an extra band on the distal long arm of chromosome 14. When looked at more closely, it turned out that the extra piece on 14 was translocated from chromosome 8 (8/14 translocation) (Fig. 2). The variant translocations were also very interesting, because in about 5% each, the same portion of chromosome 8 went to either chromosome 2 or chromosome 22. It was originally known that the immunoglobulin

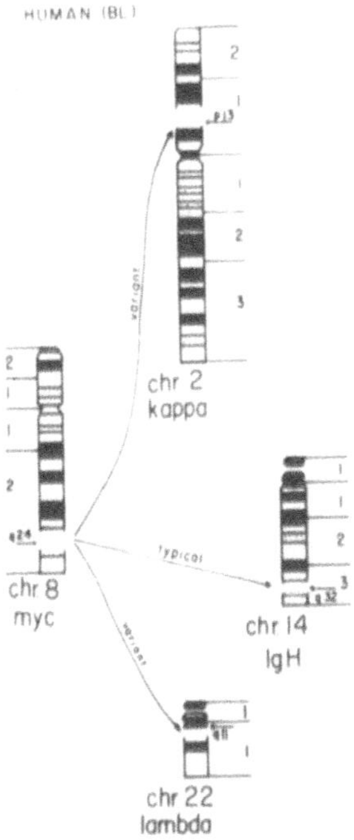

FIGURE 2. Schematic representation of typical and variant translocations involving c-myc on chromosome 8 in human Burkitt's lymphoma (BL). The typical translocation (8/14) involves the movement of c-myc to the immunoglobulin heavy chain locus (IgH) on chromosome 14. The variant translocations (8/2; 8/22) involve the movement of c-myc to either the kappa light chain on chromosome 2 or to the lambda light chain locus on chromosome 22.

heavy chain (IgH) locus was localized on chromosome 14, and later it was shown that the IgH locus was located right at the breakpoint. With the use of in situ hybridization techniques, chromosome 2 was later found to carry the kappa gene locus at the breakpoint; and chromosome 22 carries the lambda gene locus, again near the breakpoint. The only three recipient human chromosomes (14, 2, and 22), therefore, contained the three immunoglobulin gene loci, with the donor piece of chromosome 8 always being the same (reviewed in references 2 and 4). So again it was postulated that oncogene was located on chromosome 8 and that, as in the mouse, it should be c-myc. Again this was true. It should also be stressed that with the exception of c-myc similarity, there are no other homologies between human chromosome 8 and mouse chromosome 15.

The detailed molecular analysis of the c-myc oncogene then

followed. The myc oncogene has three exons. The first exon does not code for protein, and it is an unusually long leader sequence. All the coding sequences are found in the second and third exons. The virally carried v-myc, which is carried by the avian MC29 acute leukemia virus, also contains only the two coding exons. The most frequent breakpoint of the c-myc gene in mouse plasmacytomas is within the c-myc gene, and always involves the noncoding exon or its 3' intron. For some time this observation was considered important since the "decapitation" of the gene, as it was called, might have resulted in the removal of the necessary 5' regulatory sequences, resulting in the activation and transcription of the coding exons, which are always found to be highly transcribed in these B cell tumors. This has now turned out to be a more complex picture, since there are many breakpoints which occur outside the myc gene on either the 5' or 3' side. In the human situation, the variability of the breakpoint in and around the myc gene is even greater than in the mouse. There is therefore a wide variety of translocational breakpoints which are associated and compatible with the activation and increased transcription of the c-myc gene. Therefore the hypothesis that one single enhancer or promoter is responsible for the activation of c-myc is no longer tenable (reviewed in reference 5).

It is interesting, however, that in the mouse plasmacytoma system, the translocated myc gene faces the switch alpha region of the nonproductively rearranged allele of chromosome 12. In the human the translocated myc gene is most commonly found in the switch mu region of chromosome 14. Most of the mouse plasmacytomas produce IgA, and most of the human Burkitt's lymphomas make IgM, again with some exceptions. This is, however, a pseudofunction correlation, because a broken immunoglobulin heavy chain locus will not make functional immunoglobulin; it is the allele on the other chromosome that codes for the functional immunoglobulin protein. Why this pseudofunction correlation exists is, in itself, an interesting question. It tells us something about the tandem bahavior of the two chromosomes in normal DNA rearrangement during B-cell differentiation. It is thought that this DNA rearrangement during B-cell differentiation is the mechanism which provides the sensitive and vulnerable hot spot to which the translocation can occur.

From these initial observations, another set of questions can then be asked. First of all, are these myc translocations essential for generating B-cell tumors? How do the translocations arise? How do they act? What is their position within the chain of progression of events? And finally, are there functional and analogous translocations in other systems?

Firstly, it can be said that the myc translocation appears to be an essential step in genesis of B cell tumors, since in EBV-positive or EBV-negative Burkitt's lymphoma/leukemia, the association of myc transloctions is 100% at the moment (provided we throw out the atypical BJAB cell line). Although the association of myc translocations in mouse plasmacytoma is only 85%, as determined by karyotype analysis, we are now appreciating subtle molecular differences in myc rearrangements, which are not detectable at the karyotype level. It is therefore widely held that these translocations are an essential event in the development of these B cell tumors.

How do myc translocations arise? The first question to ask is, why should they be present in mouse plasmacytoma and Burkitt's lymphoma, which are different B cell tumors? Mouse plasmacytoma is a mature plasma cell, while Burkitt's lymphoma is an immature B cell, found much earlier in differentiation than a mature plasma cell. The only common denominator between these two diverse B cell tumors is the long preneoplastic latency period. In Burkitt's lymphoma, B cells are stimulated by the combination of Epstein-Barr virus (EBV) and chronic malaria. In the mouse plasmacytoma, B cells are stimulated by mineral oil-induced granuloma in the peritoneal cavity. These preneoplastic B cells persist for long periods of time and are continuously being stimulated to divide, which increases the risk of genetic abberation with each division.

How does the translocation act? The cellular myc gene in nonneoplastic B cells is known to be switched on during the first 2-4 hours after mitogenic stimulation and is then very quickly switched off.[6] It is logical to hypothesize that persistent activation and expression of the myc gene, as observed in neoplastic B cells, would result in persistent entry into the cell cycle with increased susceptibility to the action of growth factors. In time, the neoplastic B cells would become growth factor-independent and autonomous. It would therefore seem that the cellular myc gene plays a key event in the regulation of entry of the cell into the cell cycle. Since immunoglobulin genes are being transcribed during the entire cell cycle, and since the translocated myc gene comes under the influence of the immunoglobulin gene region, the myc gene is therefore transcribed during the entire cell cycle. The available data is in support of this concept. It should be stressed at this point that the myc protein, although quantitatively increased, appears to be qualitatively normal and not mutated.

If it is true that myc controls an early event in cell division, then its activation should be capable of turning normal cells into neoplastic cells, irrespective of the cell type. It is interesting to note that the virally carried myc is the only known retroviral oncogene that can induce all three major types of tumors--sarcomas, carcinomas and leukemias. One would also expect from the available data that the turn on of c-myc should be able to influence the early or late development of all three types of tumors. This appears to be true, since myc sequences are highly amplified in the latter stages of colorectal carcinomas, some hepatomas, some plasma cell leukemias, and some small cell lung carcinomas. Interestingly, the amplification of myc in lung carcinomas can either be with regard to c-myc or the cousin of c-myc, n-myc, which was picked up from a gene library by sequence homology, and which otherwise is not known to be active as an oncogene. This is also interesting since n-myc is greatly amplified in the latter stages of neuroblastoma.[7]

Do analogous translocations occur in other systems as well? The best example is the case of the Philadelphia chromosome in patients with chronic myelogenous leukemia (CML), where it has been shown that c-abl oncogene, which is located at the tip of chromosome 9, moves over to chromosome 22.[8] What about the variant translocations which occur in 10% of patients with CML? It is known from in situ hybridization experiments that the variant translocations are really three-way translocations involving the tip of 9 moving to 22 in all cases investigated so far. This molecular change is too small to be evident on karyotype analysis.

In conclusion, a possible generalized and unifying hypothesis would be the presence of a highly transcriptionally active recipient chromosomal locus which is associated with the regular need for DNA rearrangement during normal differentiation. It would be by this generalized mechanism that a translocated oncogene would come under the influence of a transcriptionally active recipient chromosomal locus.

REFERENCES

1. Klein G. 1981. The role of gene dosage and genetic transpositions in carcinogenesis. Nature 294:313-319.
2. Klein G. 1983. Specific chromosomal translocations and the genesis of B cell-derived tumors in mice and men. Cell 32:311-315.
3. Hayward WS, Neel BG Astrin SW. 1981. Activation of a cellular onc gene by promoter insertion in ALV-induced lymphoid leukosis. Nature 290:475-480.
4. Croce CM, Tsujimoto Y, Erikson J, Nowell P. 1984. Chromosomal translocations and B cell neoplasia. Lab Invest 51:258-267.
5. Perry RP. 1983. Consequences of myc invasion of immunoglobulin loci: facts and speculations. Cell 33:647-649.
6. Kelly K, Cochran BH, Stiles CD, Leder P. 1983. Cell-specific regulation of the c-myc gene by lymphocyte mitogens and platelet derived growth factor. Cell 35:603-610, 1983.
7. Kohl NE, Gee CE, Alt FW. 1984. Activated expression of the N-myc gene in human neuroblastomas and related tumors. Science 226: 1335-1336.
8. deKlein G, vanKessel AD, Grosveld G, Bartram CR, Hagemeijer A, Bootsma D, Spurr NK, Heisterkamp N, Groffen J, Stephenson JR. 1982. A cellular oncogene is translocated to the Philadelphia chromosome in chronic myelocytic leukemia. Nature 300:765-767.

MOLECULAR ANALYSIS OF THE HUMAN INTERLEUKIN-2 RECEPTOR

WARNER C. GREENE, JOEL M. DEPPER, GERALD R. CRABTREE, STUART RUDIKOFF, JANET PUMPHREY, RICHARD J. ROBB, MARTIN KRONKE, PENNY SVETLIK, NANCY J. PEFFER, THOMAS A. WALDMANN, AND WARREN J. LEONARD

1. INTRODUCTION

Complete expression of the human immune response requires the generation of activated T cells[1]. This activation sequence is initiated by an interaction of antigen with specific receptors present on the membrane of resting T cells. This receptor-ligand interaction, in the presence of macrophage derived interleukin-1 (IL-1), then triggers the production of interleukin-2 (IL-2, previously designated T cell growth factor)[2,3]. IL-2 is a well-characterized 14,500 dalton glycoprotein which promotes T cell proliferation following binding to specific high affinity IL-2 membrane receptors[4-6]. However, unlike receptors for antigen, IL-2 receptors are not expressed by resting T cells, but like IL-2, are synthesized following antigen activation. The interaction of IL-2 with its inducible receptor results in T cell proliferation and expansion of the antigen reactive T cell clone and culminates in the emergence of T cells mediating helper, suppressor, and cytotoxic T cell function. Thus, both the specificity and magnitude of the T cell immune response is in large measure controlled at the level of IL-2 receptor expression.

IL-2 cDNAs have been isolated and expressed in prokaryotic and eukaryotic cells[7-8]. The human IL-2 gene has been cloned, completely sequenced, and localized to chromosome 4[9,10]. Further, post-translational processing including the formation of a single disulfide bond and addition of 0-linked carbohydrate to the third amino acid (threonine) has been detected[4].

We have previously demonstrated that monoclonal anti-Tac antibody, prepared by Uchiyama and Waldmann[11], recognizes the human IL-2 receptor[12-16]. We have used this monoclonal antibody to biochemically characterize this receptor[12,13,17]. The human

IL-2 receptor isolated from normal activated T cells is a glycosylated, sulfated, and phosphorylated structure containing intrachain disulfide bonds with an apparent M_r of 55,000[13,17]. The protein backbone of this receptor has an M_r of 33,000 and is cotranslationally processed by the addition of N-linked carbohydrate to yield two precursor forms (M_r 35,000 and 37,000). These N-glycosylated precursors are exported to the Golgi apparatus where additional post-translational processing occurs including the addition of O-linked carbohydrate and sialic acid. We now describe the purification of IL-2 receptor protein, and the isolation and expression of cDNAs encoding this receptor. A more complete description of these studies is presented in reference 18.

2. PURIFICATION AND DETERMINATION OF THE N-TERMINAL AMINO ACID SEQUENCE OF THE HUMAN IL-2 RECEPTOR

To facilitate the isolation of significant quantities of IL-2 receptor protein, we elected to utilize a human T cell line, HUT 102B2, which is infected with the human T cell leukemia-lymphoma virus-type 1 (HTLV-1)[19]. These cells and other cell lines infected with this human retrovirus constitutively express large numbers of IL-2 receptors[20]. Monoclonal anti-Tac antibody was covalently coupled to cyanogen bromide activated Sepharose 4B beads and used as an immunoaffinity support. HUT 102B2 cells were solubilized in NP-40 detergent and clarified cellular extracts were passed over a control monoclonal UPC10 antibody column and then over the anti-Tac column. The anti-Tac column was washed with buffers of differing ionic strength and the retained protein then eluted in 2.5% acetic acid. A silver stain of eluted protein electrophoresed on an 8.75% SDS-polyacrylamide gel is shown in Figure 1. The size of this protein is identical to that of the IL-2 receptor identified by anti-Tac immunoprecipitation of ^{35}S-methionine labeled or surface iodinated HUT 102B2 cells. Furthermore, the eluted protein retained the capacity to bind IL-2.

The sequence of the 29 N-terminal amino acids of the IL-2 receptor was determined by automated Edman degradations in a gas phase microsequencer (100-250 picomoles per analysis). In

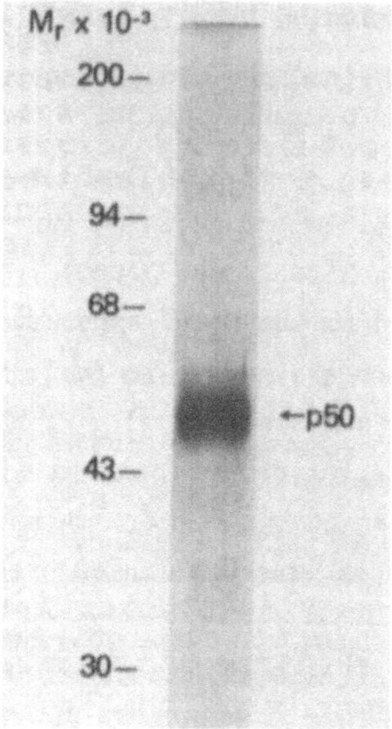

FIGURE 1. Silver stain of the HUT 102B2 human IL-2 receptor purified by immunoaffinity chromatography using monoclonal anti-Tac antibody. Migration of known molecular weight markers is indicated.

addition, certain positions were confirmed or identified by sequencing receptor biosynthetically labeled with radioactive amino acids in a spinning cup apparatus.

3. ISOLATION OF cDNAs ENCODING THE HUMAN IL-2 RECEPTOR

A 17 base oligonucleotide probe with 64 fold degeneracy was synthesized based on the amino acid sequence of residues 3-8. Following end-labeling with ^{32}P using polynucleotide kinase, this probe was used to screen a lambda gt10 cDNA library prepared with oligo dT selected HUT 102B2 mRNA. The entire cDNA library contained 2.4 million recombinant clones with inserts ranging in size from 500 bp to several kilobases. Following amplification of the library, approximately 200,000 phage clones were screened under conditions of hybridization and washing which yielded discrete signals on Northern blots of HUT 102B2 mRNA. Following serial screening, we isolated 11 candidate clones for the IL-2

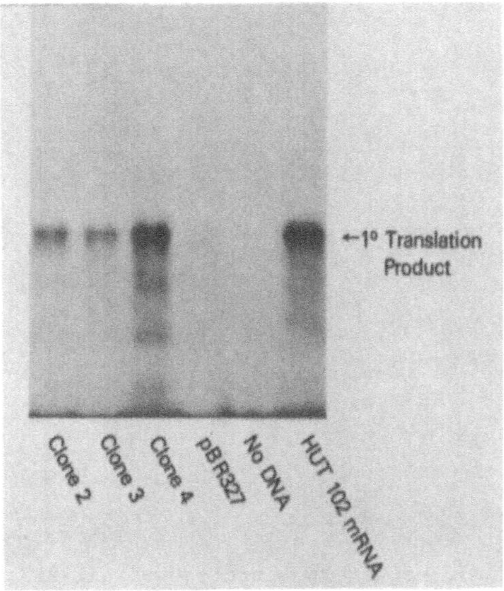

FIGURE 2. Selective hybridization of mRNA by candidate IL-2 receptor cDNAs. Selected mRNA was translated in a wheat germ lysate cell-free translation system and immunoprecipitated with a monospecific rabbit anti-IL-2 receptor antiserum prepared by immunization with purified receptor protein. Previous studies had demonstrated that monoclonal anti-Tac did not precipitate the primary translation product of the IL-2 receptor.

---

receptor. Inserts from these 11 recombinant phage clones ranged in size from 0.9 to 2.4 kilobases.

Inserts from three of the candidate phage clones were then subcloned into pBR322 (designated pIL-2R2, pIL-2R3, and pIL-2R4) and evaluated for their capacity to selectively hybridize IL-2 receptor mRNA from HUT 102B2 cells[21]. As shown in Figure 2, linearized plasmids containing cDNA inserts from each of the three candidate IL-2 receptor clones bound to nitrocellulose filters successfully hybridized mRNA which when translated and immunoprecipitated revealed a protein identical in size to the primary translation product for the IL-2 receptor. In contrast, filters which contained no DNA or control pBR327 DNA did not retain IL-2 receptor mRNA. We felt these data indicated that we had isolated IL-2 receptor associated clones but did not constitute formal proof that the receptor was cloned.

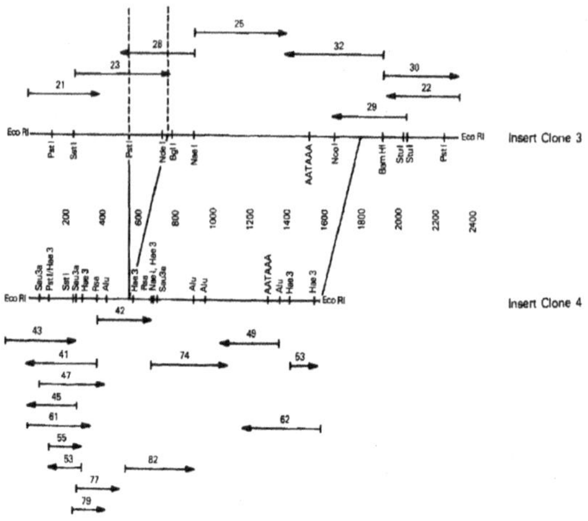

FIGURE 3. Restriction map and M13 sequencing strategy of pIL-2R3 and pIL-2R4. The region of 216 bp present in clone 3 but absent in clone 4 is indicated.

We next restricted and subcloned each of the three cDNA inserts into M13 bacteriophage and determined their complete nucleotide sequence by the dideoxynucleotide chain termination method of Sanger[22]. The sequencing strategies and restriction maps for pIL-2R3 and pIL-2R4 is shown in Figure 3. All sequences were analyzed on an IMB 360 computer using the program of Queen and Korn[24]. Each of the cDNA inserts contained a single long open reading frame, including a 5' sequence of 87 nucleotides which precisely matched the 29 amino acids determined by amino acid sequencing thus confirming their relationship to the human IL-2 receptor. However, further comparison of the sequences of pIL-2R3 and pIL-2R4 revealed an important difference. Clone 3 contained a segment of 216 base pairs which was missing from clone 4. This region was within the protein coding region and was flanked by classical mRNA donor and acceptor splicing sites (AGGT)[24]. Thus, it seemed likely that we had cloned cDNAs representative of a spliced and unspliced IL-2 receptor mRNA. Splicing of this internal segment did not result in a frame shift thus the predicted proteins shared common amino and carboxy sequences and only differed by the presence or absence of a central region composed of 72 amino acids. Further, we were left with the dilemma of whether only one or both of the respective mRNAs encoded the IL-2 receptor. To address this question, we used the cDNAs to direct the synthesis of their respective proteins. An expression vector, pCEXV-1 (generously provided by Drs. Ron Germain and Jim Miller, NIH), which contain SV40 promoter and enhancer sequences was used for this purpose. The "spliced" (clone 4) and "unspliced" (clone 3) cDNAs were inserted into this vector in the proper orientation and then transfected by calcium phosphate precipitation into COS-1 cells. The presence of T antigen in these cells promotes high level expression of protein under the control of the SV40 promoter. Following 48 hours of culture, the COS cells were assayed for the presence of IL-2 receptors using radiolabeled purified IL-2 and anti-Tac. As shown in Figure 4, COS cells transfected with clone 3, the unspliced cDNA, expressed surface receptors recognized both by IL-2 and anti-Tac. In contrast, the spliced cDNA did not direct the synthesis of a protein capable of binding IL-2 or anti-Tac. In view of these data, we screened the remaining eight cDNA clones for the presence or absence of this internal segment. Each of these eight cDNAs appeared to correspond to unspliced forms of IL-2 mRNA. As we had only a single spliced cDNA, we were concerned that this clone could be the result of an artifact occuring during the cloning procedure. However, S1 nuclease protection assays utilizing an M13 subclone which bridges the spliceable segment clearly indicated that this spliced IL-2 receptor mRNA is present not only in HUT 102B2 cells but other HTLV infected leukemic cells as well as normal activated T cells. These data raise the interesting possibility that IL-2 receptor expression may not only be regulated at the level of initiation of transcription but as well through changes in the post-transcriptional splicing.

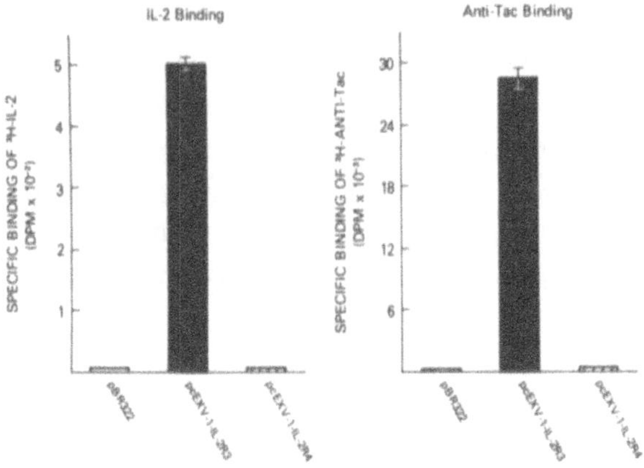

FIGURE 4. Expression of IL-2 receptor cDNAs in COS-1 cells and detection of IL-2 receptors by binding of purified radiolabeled IL-2 and anti-Tac.

4. SOUTHERN AND NORTHERN BLOT ANALYSIS OF THE IL-2 RECEPTOR

To evaluate whether the IL-2 receptor was encoded by a single structural gene or alternatively existed as a member of a multiple gene family, genomic DNA from three different sources was restricted with EcoRl or BamHl, transferred to nitrocellulose, and hybridized with a probe composed of the first 700 nucleotides of the IL-2 receptor. As shown in Panel A of Figure 5, very simple banding patterns were observed suggesting the presence of a single structural gene.

We next studied expression of IL-2 receptor mRNA in varying lymphoid populations. As shown in panel B of Figure 5, unstimulated peripheral blood lymphocytes contained no detectable IL-2 receptor mRNA. As the IL-2 receptor is a T cell activation antigen, this result was not surprising. Activation of these cells with PHA and phorbol myristate acetate (PMA) resulted in the expression of two different mRNAs which hybridized to the IL-2 receptor cDNA probe. Similar sized mRNAs were present in HTLV-1 infected HUT 102B2 cells. The acute lymphocytic leukemic T cell lines, CEM and HSB-2, which do not display IL-2 receptors

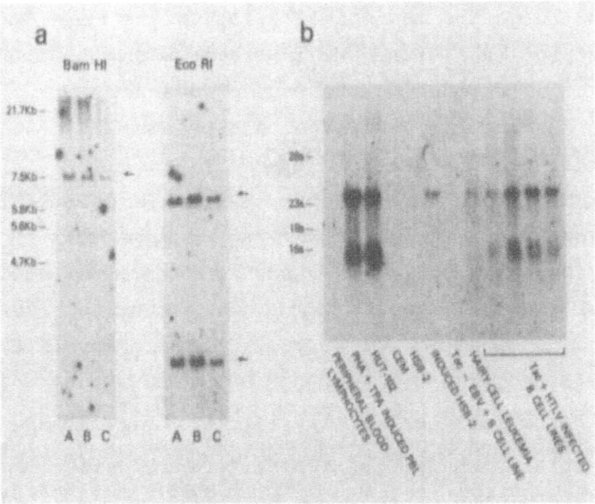

FIGURE 5. Panel A: Southern blot analysis of EcoR1 and BamH1 restricted human DNA probed with an IL-2 receptor cDNA composed of the initial 700 base pairs of the receptor. Subsequent blots with full length cDNA probes have revealed 5 EcoR1 fragments and 2 BamH1 fragments. Panel B: Northern blot analysis of poly A^+ mRNA from varying lymphoid cell lines hybridized with an IL-2 receptor cDNA.

on their cell surfaces, did not contain IL-2 receptor mRNA. However, we have previously demonstrated that induction of HSB-2 cells with PMA resulted in expression of the Tac antigen (monoclonal anti-Tac antibody binds to both high and low affinity IL-2 receptors)[25]. Similarly, IL-2 receptor mRNA was detectable in HSB-2 cells induced with PMA although the larger mRNA form was considerably more prevalent. In addition to T cells, we analyzed expression of IL-2 receptor mRNA in varying B cell populations. One EBV transformed B cell line which did not react with anti-Tac did not contain IL-2 receptor mRNA. In contrast, Hairy Cell Leukemia cells which display the Tac antigen[26] contained detectable IL-2 receptor mRNA. These leukemia cells are B cells as indicated by effective rearrangement of heavy and light chain Ig genes[26]. Recently, it has been possible to establish long-term B cell lines infected with HTLV-1 without concomitant EBV infection.

We observed that each of these lines expressed IL-2 receptor mRNA.

We next attempted to define the molecular basis for the difference in IL-2 receptor mRNA size. We initially were concerned that the two mRNAs might differ due to presence or absence of the spliceable internal segment. To evaluate this possibility. we prepared DNA from this region (Pst-NdeI fragment) and used it to probe HUT 102B2 mRNA. Both IL-2 receptor mRNAs hybridized with this probe (data not shown). In view of the expression results, this finding suggested that both forms of the mRNA were functional. This suggestion was confirmed by isolation of the primary translation product for the IL-2 receptor in translations of mRNA from both hybridizing regions.

Further analysis of the sequence of the IL-2 receptor cDNAs suggested a possible explanation for the two differently sized mRNAs. Distal to the end of the protein coding region we detected the presence of a polyadenylation signal sequence (AATAAA). In most eucaryotic mRNAs, polyadenylation normally occurs approximately 12-18 residues downstream from this signal sequence. However, polyadenylation did not occur in our cDNA clone. Thus, we hypothesized that use of this polyadenylation site would generate the short form of the IL-2 receptor mRNA while use of a more distal polyadenylation signal sequence would produce the larger mRNA. To test this hypothesis, we prepared a 3' probe which consisted of sequences distal to the proximal polyadenylation signal sequence (NcoI-EcoR1 fragment) and used this fragment to probe HUT 102B2 mRNA. As shown in Figure 6, this probe only hybridized to the large form of the IL-2 receptor mRNA. These data indicate that the two differently sized IL-2 receptor mRNAs are generated through the use of different polyadenylation signal sequences.

5. AMINO ACID SEQUENCE OF THE HUMAN IL-2 RECEPTOR

Determination of the complete cDNA sequence of the IL-2 receptor allowed us to deduce the amino acid sequence of the protein. As shown in Figure 7, the IL-2 receptor is composed of

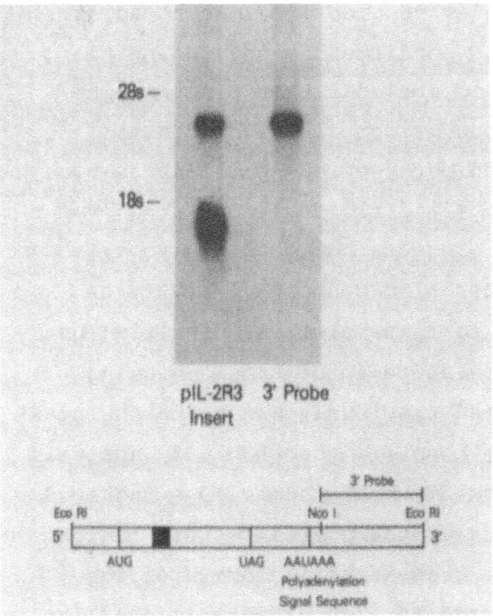

FIGURE 6. Full-length and 3' IL-2 receptor cDNA probes hybridized to HUT 102B2 mRNA indicating that the two IL-2 receptor mRNAs differ in the polyadenylation signal sequence utilized.

−21 Met Asp Ser Tyr Leu Leu Met Trp Gly Leu Leu Thr Phe Ile Met Val Pro Gly Cys Gln
−1 Ala Glu Leu Cys Asp Asp Asp Pro Pro Glu Ile Pro His Ala Thr Phe Lys Ala Met Ala
20 Tyr Lys Glu Gly Thr Met Leu Asn Cys Glu Cys Lys Arg Gly Phe Arg Arg Ile Lys Ser
40 Gly Ser Leu Tyr Met Leu Cys Thr Gly Asn Ser Ser His Ser Ser Trp Asp Asn Gln Cys
60 Gln Cys Thr Ser Ser Ala Thr Arg Asn Thr Thr Lys Gln Val Thr Pro Gln Pro Glu Glu
80 Gln Lys Glu Arg Lys Thr Thr Glu Met Gln Ser Pro Met Gln Pro Val Asp Gln Ala Ser
100 Leu Pro Gly His Cys Arg Glu Pro Pro Pro Trp Glu Asn Glu Ala Thr Glu Arg Ile Tyr
120 His Phe Val Val Gly Gln Met Val Tyr Tyr Gln Cys Val Gln Gly Tyr Arg Ala Leu His
160 Arg Gly Pro Ala Glu Ser Val Cys Lys Met Thr His Gly Lys Thr Arg Trp Thr Gln Pro
140 Gln Leu Ile Cys Thr Gly Glu Met Glu Thr Ser Gln Phe Pro Gly Glu Glu Lys Pro Gln
180 Ala Ser Pro Glu Gly Arg Pro Glu Ser Glu Thr Ser Cys Leu Val Thr Thr Thr Asp Phe
200 Gln Ile Gln Thr Glu Met Ala Ala Thr Met Glu Thr Ser Ile Phe Thr Thr Glu Tyr Gln
220 Val Ala Val Ala Gly Cys Val Phe Leu Leu Ile Ser Val Leu Leu Leu Ser Gly Leu Thr
240 Trp Gln Arg Arg Gln Arg Lys Ser Arg Arg Thr Ile 251

FIGURE 7. Deduced amino acid sequence of the human IL-2 receptor. Signal peptide, two potential N-glycosylation sites, the hydrophobic transmembrane domain, and the intracytoplasmic domain are indicated.

272 amino acids including a leader peptide of 21 amino acids. Length of the leader peptide was confirmed by sequencing the primary translation product radiolabeled with ^{35}S-methionine. The primary sequence of the receptor contains two potential N-glycosylation sites. Based on our previous pulse-chase biosynthetic studies in which we identified two N-glycosylated precursors (M_r 35,000 and 37,000) we suggest that both N-glycosylation sites are utilized. The receptor also contains 13 cysteine residues which may participate in intramolecular disulfide bonding. Migration of the radiolabeled receptor under reducing versus nonreducing conditions had previously suggested the presence of such internal disulfide bonds. Hydrophobicity analysis indicated the presence of a markedly hydrophobic 19 amino acid region near the carboxy terminus of the protein. This region almost certainly represents the transmembrane domain of the receptor. The intracytoplasmic domain is characterized by the presence of lysine and arginine residues which impart a positive charge and presumably subserve a cytoplasmic anchoring function. Further, this intracytoplasmic region is but 13 amino acids long. Thus, it would appear unlikely that this region encodes an enzymatic function. These data raise important questions regarding the mechanism by which binding of IL-2 to its receptor generates the signal leading to T cell proliferation. We have previously identified two other proteins which are coimmunoprecipitated with the M_r 55,000 protein we have cloned[12,17]. These proteins have apparent M_r's of 113,000 and 180,000 and are phosphorylated but not glycosylated nor labeled by cell surface iodination. It is possible, though unproven, that these proteins may participate in the formation of a receptor complex.

The intracytoplasmic domain also contains serine and threonine but not tyrosine phosphate acceptor sites. We have previously demonstrated that the IL-2 receptor is a phosphoprotein.

Comparison of the sequence of the IL-2 receptor to all other known DNA and protein sequences registered in the Georgetown and Los Alamos data bases revealed no significant homologies. Thus, while v-erb-b and the receptor for epidermal growth factor share striking regions of homology[27], the possible general relationship of growth factor receptors to oncogenes apparently cannot be extended to the human IL-2 receptor. The availability of cDNA probes for the human IL-2 receptor should aid in studies of IL-2 receptor structure, function, and regulation. Coupled with the availability of recombinant IL-2, study of IL-2-IL-2 receptor interactions may be performed with well-characterized purified reagents.

REFERENCES

1. Farrar JJ, Benjamin WR, Hilfiker ML, Howard M, Farrar WJ, Fuller-Farrar J. 1982. Immunol Rev 63:129.
2. Morgan DA, Ruscetti FW, Gallo RC. 1976. Science 193:1077.
3. Smith KA. 1980. Immunol Rev 51:337.
4. Robb RJ, Kutny RM, Chowdhry V. 1983. Proc Natl Acad Sci USA 80:5990.
5. Robb RJ, Munck A, Smith KA. 1981. J Exp Med 154:1455.
6. Greene WC, Robb RJ. 1984, in press. In: Contemporary Topics in Molecular Immunology, Gillis S (ed). New York, Plenum Press.
7. Taniguchi T, Matsui H, Funita T, Takaoka C, Kashima N, Yoshimoto R, Hamuro J. 1983. Nature 302:305.
8. Devos R, Paetinck G, Cheroute H, Simons G, Degrave W, Tavernier J, Remout E, Fiers W. 1983. Nucleic Acid Res 11:4307.
9. Fujita T, Takeoka C, Matsui H, Taniguchi T. 1983. Proc Natl Acad Sci USA 80:1634.
10. Holbrook NJ, Smith KA, Fornace AJ Jr, Comeau CM, Wiskocil RL, Crabtree GR. 1984. Proc Natl Acad Sci USA 81:1634.
11. Uchiyama T, Broder S, Waldmann TA. 1981. J Immunol 126:1393.
12. Leonard WJ, Depper JM, Uchiyama T, Smith KA, Waldmann TA, Greene WC. 1982. Nature 300:267.
13. Leonard WJ, Depper JM, Robb RJ, Waldmann TA, Greene WC. 1983. Proc Natl Acad Sci USA 80:6957.
14. Robb RJ, Greene WC. 1983. J Exp Med 158:1332.
15. Leonard WJ, Depper JM, Waldmann TA, Greene WC. 1984. In: Receptors and Recognition, Vol 17, Greaves M (ed). p45.
16. Depper JM, Leonard WJ, Robb RJ, Waldmann TA, Greene WC. 1983. J Immunol 131:690.
17. Leonard WJ, Depper JM, Robb RJ, Kronke M, Waldmann TA, Greene WC. 1985, in press, J Biol Chem.
18. Leonard WJ, Depper JM, Crabtree GR, Rudikoff S, Pumphrey J, Robb RJ, Kronke M, Svetlik PB, Peffer NJ, Waldmann TA, Greene WC. 1984. Nature 311:626.
19. Poiesz BJ, Ruscetti RW, Gazdar AF, Bunn PA, Minna JO, Gallo RC. 1980. Proc Natl Acad Sci USA 77:7415.
20. Depper JM, Leonard WJ, Kronke M, Waldmann TA, Greene WC. 1984. J Immunol 133:1691.
21. Maniatis T, Fritsch EF, Sambrook J. 1982. In: Molecular Cloning. Cold Spring Harbor, Cold Spring Harbor Laboratory, p330.
22. Sanger F, Coulson AR. 1975. J Mol Biol 94:414.
23. Queen CL, Korn CJ. 1980. J Meth Enzym 65:595.

24. Breathnach R, Benoist C, O'Hare K, Gannon F, Chambon P. 1978. Proc Natl Acad Sci USA 75:4853.
25. Greene WC, Robb RJ, Depper JM, Leonard WJ, Drogula C, Svetlik PB, Wong-Staal F, Gallo RC, Waldmann TA, Greene WC. 1984. J Immunol 133:1042.
26. Korsmeyer SJ, Greene WC, Cossman J, Hsu SM, Jensen JP, Neckers LM, Marshall SL, Bakhshi A, Depper JM, Leonard WJ, Jaffe ES, Waldmann TA. 1983. Proc Natl Acad Sci USA 80:4522.
27. Downard J, et al. 1984. Nature 307:521.

DNA REARRANGEMENTS AS UNIQUE MOLECULAR MARKERS OF CLONALITY, CELLULAR LINEAGE, DIFFERENTIATION, AND TRANSLOCATION

S.J. KORSMEYER, A. BAKHSHI, K.A. SIMINOVITCH, AND J.J. WRIGHT

The demonstration that clinically and histologically distinct lymphoid neoplasms could be assigned to stages of B or T cell development was of immense importance in furthering our understanding of the biology of these malignancies[1,2]. This has been accomplished predominantly by utilizing cell surface markers associated with various developmental stages of B or T cell maturation. In addition, the demonstration that certain neoplasms were a monoclonal proliferation was of great conceptual importance in understanding their pathogenesis[3]. Despite a large number of lineage-associated cell surface markers, it is still frequently impossible to conclusively classify a lymphoid neoplasm as B or T cell in origin. This is often due to the admixture of large numbers of non-neoplastic cells with the neoplastic cells in a lymphomatous tissue. Furthermore, other malignancies may be at a stage of differentiation prior to the expression of any lineage-restricted cell surface antigen. Beyond this, the determination of clonality in lymphoid neoplasms has been practically limited to the mature B cell malignancies that display the presence of but one light-chain isotype, κ or λ.

Because of the frequent inadequacies in assigning the cellular lineage, stage of differentiation, and clonality of lymphoid neoplasms, we have pursued a molecular genetic approach. Specifically we have utilized the DNA rearrangements which assemble the gene subsegments for antigen-specific receptors in B cells as well as T cells as molecular markers which are unique to individual neoplasms.

The rearrangements of Ig genes and the β chain of the T cell antigen-specific receptor have proven not only to be lineage associated, but are also extremely sensitive markers for clonality[4]. They have resolved issues concerning the cellular lineage commitment, clonality, and stage of differentiation of lymphoid neoplasms that were uncertain by phenotypic analysis alone. In addition, further recombinations of especially the Ig gene loci have been defined which contribute directly to the malignant phenotype. This latter type of rearrangement occurs between non-homologous chromosomes and translocates a cellular oncogene into an Ig gene locus and its influence[5,6].

DNA Rearrangements Which Assemble Ig Genes Create Unique Clonal Markers

The mechanism which activates an Ig gene generates a clonal marker specific to that particular B cell. This is the result of the process of DNA rearrangement which moves and combines the separated gene segments which encode the final Ig molecule. As shown in Figure 1, of the multitude of available variable κ regions (V_κ), one is juxtaposed with one of five joining (J_κ) segments[7,8]. These combined V_κ/J_κ segments encode the entire

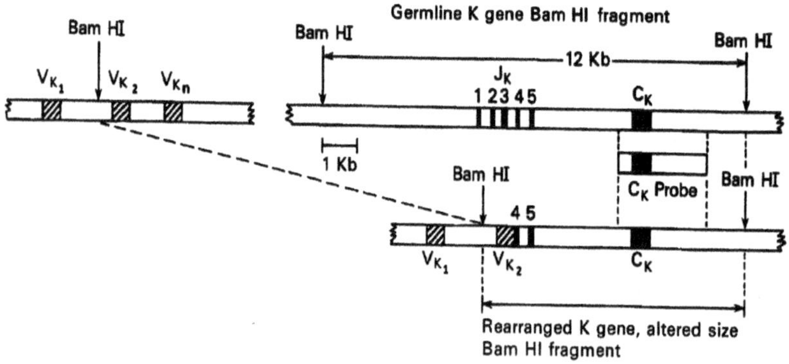

FIGURE 1. A germline and rearranged κ gene allele. One of many variable (V_κ) segments is rearranged to a single joining ($J_\kappa 4$) segment. This rearrangement introduces as new 5' BamHI site so that the BamHI restriction endonuclease fragment recognized by the constant κ (C_κ) probe differs in size from the germline fragment.

variable portion of the molecule. This rearranged κ allele is then transcribed and the $V_κ/J_κ$ and constant ($C_κ$) information are spliced together at an RNA level. It is, however, the process of DNA rearrangement which creates a molecular marker that is unique to an individual cell (Fig. 1). The act of V/J joining introduces a new restriction endonuclease site and thus alters the size of the restriction fragment containing the κ gene. Therefore, a rearranged Ig gene is found on a different sized DNA restriction fragment as compared to its germline or embryonic form. A polyclonal population of normal B cells is comprised of many different cells which possess numerous different Ig gene rearrangements; none of the rearranged genes in this collective population will be discernible by Southern blot analysis because they fall below the threshhold of detection[9]. In contrast, a monoclonal expansion of B cells represents the progeny of an original single cell and possesses multiple copies of the same DNA rearrangement unique to that cell. Such clonal DNA rearrangements are detectable even if the clonal B cell represents only 1-5% of the total cells present[4,10]. Thus lineage-associated DNA rearrangements serve as sensitive as well as specific clonal markers.

Ig Gene Patterns in Mature B-Cell Malignancies and Non-B Cell Neoplasms

Mature B cells must possess a rearranged heavy (H) and light (L) chain Ig gene responsible for their cell surface Ig. Over 40 cases of chronic lymphocytic leukemia, Waldenström's macroglobulinemia, multiple myeloma, B cell follicular and diffuse lymphomas, Burkitt lymphoma, and Epstein-Barr virus transformed normal B cell lines have displayed clonal H plus L chain rearrangements. Roughly 60% of these tumors produce κ light chain, while 40% produce λ light chain. Of note, κ-producing B cells displayed at least one κ gene rearrangement, while they retained their λ genes in the germline form (Fig. 2). In striking contrast, λ-producing B cells, while displaying the obligate λ rearrangement, had surprisingly rearranged or deleted their κ genes[11]. This proved to result from an ordered sequence of

L chain genes in man in which · rearrangements preceded · (Fig. 2)[9,12].

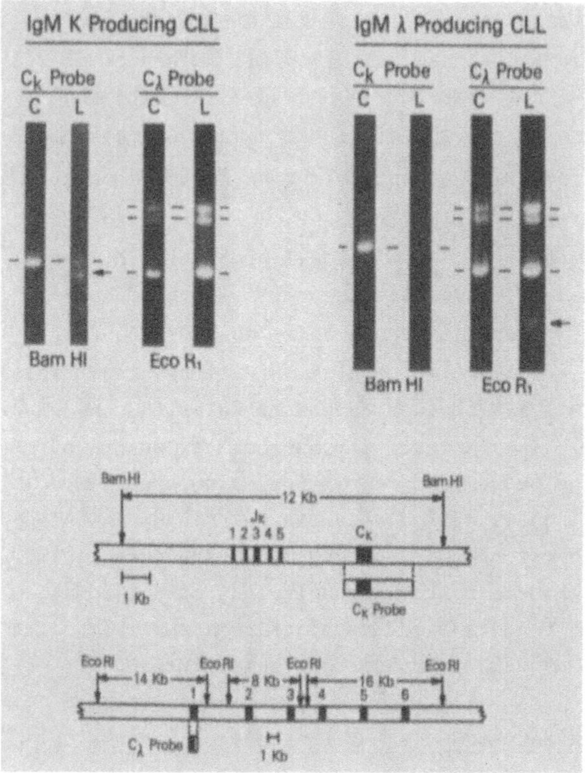

FIGURE 2. L chain genes in · and ` producing B cell chronic lymphocytic leukemia (L) as compared to their fibroblasts (C). A rearranged · gene (arrow) is present in the · -CLL while its · genes are in the germline form (dash marks). In contrast the `-CLL reveals a loss of · genes. Lower schematics reveal probes and restriction maps.

In contrast to the B cell malignancies, all T cell neoplasms we have examined have retained germline · and ` L chain genes. Furthermore, most of the T cell malignancies (23/25) also displayed germline H chain genes[4]. Similarly, malignancies of non-lymphoid hematopoietic cells including acute myelogenous leukemia, acute and chronic myeloid phases of chronic myelogenous leukemia, promyelocytic, monocytic, and histiocyte-like cells all retained germline L-chain genes and usually H-chain genes[4]. Thus, while H chain Ig gene rearrangement can occasionally spill over into other lineages, L chain rearrangements as later steps in development appear not to. Therefore, the simultaneous presence of a rearranged H plus L chain gene is a highly B cell restricted marker.

Non-T, Non-B Acute Lymphoblastic Leukemias are a Developmental Series of B-Cell Precursors

The "non-T, non-B" form of acute lymphoblastic leukemia (ALL) was of previously uncertain cellular origin because these cells lacked T cell surface antigens and also failed to display surface Ig. Analysis of their Ig genes proved that while they lacked mature cell surface markers, these leukemias reflected serial stages of B cell precursor development[12,13,14]. All cases examined have shown Ig H chain gene rearrangements. Approximately 60% of these ALLs retain germline L chain genes. This provided the first evidence in man that H chain gene rearrangements precede L chain gene rearrangements. In 40% of these pre-B cell ALLs which have progressed to L chain rearrangement there is also evidence for a κ before λ order to L chain recombination. What we observed was that cells which had rearranged or deleted their κ genes still had germline λ genes. In contrast the pre-B cells which had moved onto λ gene rearrangement uniformly had no remaining germline κ genes, having deleted them[12,13]. Thus the Ig gene pattern in these ALLs not only revealed their pre-B cell commitment, but also told us of a developmental cascade of Ig gene rearrangements in which H chain genes preceded L, and κ rearranged before λ.

Coordinate with this hierarchy of Ig gene rearrangements, we found a sequential expression of cell surface antigens (Fig. 3)[13,14]. The very earliest identifiable B cell precursors displayed H chain gene rearrangement and HLA-DR together with B_4, a B cell restricted antigen reported by Nadler et al.[15]. Later in differentiation B cell precursors add the common acute lymphoblastic leukemia antigen (CALLA) and subsequently rearrange κ or λ L chain genes. At a variable time of development the maturing pre-B cells add yet another B cell restricted antigen, B_1 (Fig. 3)[16]. This coordinate sequence of genetic and phenotypic markers has not only advanced our understanding of pre-B cell differentiation, but is providing an important means of subclassifying these leukemias based on their stage of maturational arrest.

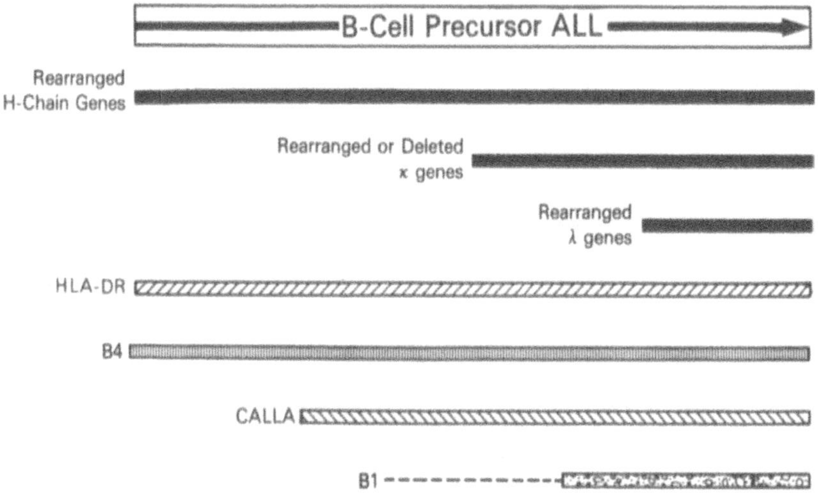

FIGURE 3. Coordinate sequence of Ig gene rearrangements and cell surface antigens in pre-B cell acute lymphoblastic leukemia. HLA-DR and B_4 antigens precede the expression of the common acute lymphoblastic leukemia antigen (CALLA) and L chain rearrangement. The B_1 antigen is added at a variable time.

Antigen-Specific Receptor Genes as Rearranging Determinants in T Cell Neoplasms

The determination that Ig genes were usually retained in their germline form within most T cells suggested that the antigen-specific receptor present on these T cells was not encoded by the Ig genes. Recently, genes for the β and candidate genes for the α chain of the heterodimeric structure comprising the T cell antigen receptor have been cloned by the groups of Davis, Mak, and Tonegawa[17-20]. The β chain gene is the best characterized and is an entirely separate gene complex from Ig and is located on chromosome 7. However, it has discontinuous gene subsegments of two constant region genes (C_1 and C_2) and each of these has associated diversity (D_1 and D_2) and joining (J_1 and J_2) regions and a set of variable (V) regions has been identified (Fig. 4). Similar to the Ig genes, the T cell β chain gene is activated by rearrangements which combine D to J segments or create a complete V/D/J complex. Due to a clever orientation of the recombinatorial signals which flank these genes, the V_1 and D_1 cluster of segments appear capable of using the second (J_2) as well as the initial (J_1) set of joining segments. Such a capability markedly augments the amount of diversity that can be generated by recombinatorial shuffling alone (Fig. 4).

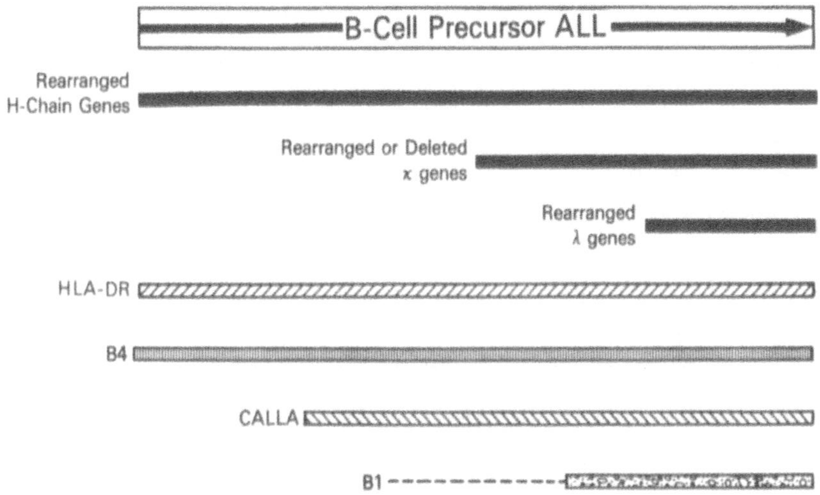

FIGURE 4. The human β chain gene of the heterodimeric T cell antigen receptor has two constant regions (C_1 and C_2) and each has its own joining (J_1 and J_2) and diversity (D_1 and D_2) segments. Variable (V) segments also exist. The spacing of the recombinatorial signals flanking these segments allows numerous recombinations markedly augmenting diversity.

The β chain genes (CT_β) must rearrange in any T cell which bears an antigen-specific receptor. This rearrangement, therefore, provides a unique molecular marker for clonal populations of T cells. This is of tremendous importance as there were no routinely available clonal markers for T cell malignancies previously. The rearrangement of the α and β chain genes within

T cells is permitting us to answer all of the issues within T cell neoplasms that were resolved by an analysis of Ig gene rearrangements in B cell neoplasms.

Detection of Clonal B Cells Within Lesions of Mixed Cellularity

The presence of Ig gene rearrangements has been instrumental in revealing that non-T, non-B ALLs and the lymphoid blast crisis phases of CML[21,22] are in reality clonal expansions of B cell precursors. Similarly the leukemic cells of Hairy Cell Leukemia proved to represent a mature B cell stage with the appropriately rearranged, switched, and expressed Ig genes[23]. The application of molecular markers has perhaps made an even greater impact upon our classification and understanding of solid lymphoid neoplasms.

A molecular approach has been crucial in classifying the cellular origin of a number of lymphomas, but particularly those with mixed cellularity. Our attention was directed to several lymphomas which contained a predominance of T cells and small numbers of B cells (Table 1)[4]. Because DNA rearrangements of Ig or β chain T cell receptor genes are extremely

Table 1. Monoclonal B-cell populations within some lymphomas with predominant T-cells.

	B cell	T cell	Surface Ig			Ig Genes
	B1	Lyt 3	H-Chain	κ	λ	T-cell Receptor Gene
Diffuse mixed Cell lymphoma	13%	73%	(-)	(-)	(-)	J_H Rearranged C_κ Rearranged CT_β Germline
Follicular and Diffuse mixed Cell Lymphoma	26%	89%	None Predominant (G 5%, A 23%, M 28%, D14%)	(-)	(-)	J_H Rearranged C_λ Rearranged CT_β Germline

sensitive as well as specific, they can detect clonal populations if they constitute only 1-5% of the total cells present. Table 1 reveals two dramatic instances of lymph node biopsies with a predominance of T cells (73-89%) and a minority of B cells with no cell surface Ig isotype predominance. However, these lesions possessed clonally rearranged H plus L chain Ig genes and retained a germline CT_β gene. This molecular analysis established that these are really clonal B cell lymphomas with an infiltrate of polyclonal T cells (Table 1).

The diagnostic choice between benign and malignant lymphoid proliferations in the setting of an immunodeficient host is frequently difficult based on histologic grounds alone. In this setting the demonstration of clonality usually based on the presence of a single surface Ig L chain (κ or λ) has been an important diagnostic aid favoring malignancy. One such difficult differential diagnosis is shown in Figure 5 where a tissue biopsy from a child with Wiskott-Aldrich syndrome and enlarging lymphadenopathy was felt to be more consistent with atypical follicular hyperplasia than with lymphoma. Compatible with this, surface marker analysis of cellular populations revealed the presence of both κ and λ bearing cells and many Lyt 3-positive T cells. However, DNA analysis detected a minority population of clonal B cells possessing rearranged H and L chain genes (Fig. 5)[4]. Thus, despite the heterogeneity within this lymph node a clonal population of B cells did exist! While this might represent the early detection of a malignancy, it was also possible that this expansion of B cells was still under some regulatory control. The specific DNA rearrangements observed did provide a unique clonal marker unique to these cells which enabled us to follow their natural history. This patient later expired from infectious causes and at autopsy showed no evidence of lymphoma. Thus, while Ig gene and CT_β gene rearrangements are sensitive detectors of clonality, they are in and of themselves not tantamount to a verdict of malignancy. As we will explore other types of rearrangements that occur within tumors may be much more specific for malignancy.

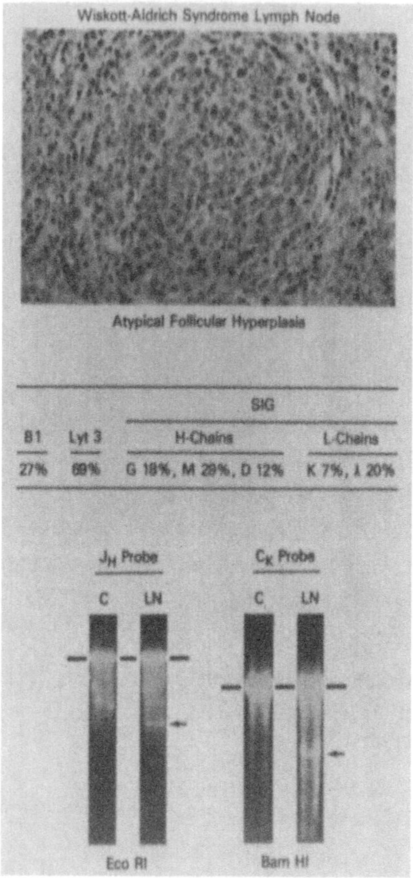

FIGURE 5. Lymph node (LN) biopsy from a patient with Wiskott-Aldrich syndrome read as atypical follicular hyperplasia. Phenotypic markers revealed a mixed lymphoid population but DNA from the LN revealed a clonal rearrangement of H and L chain genes (arrows) in a subpopulation of the cells.

Clonal Evolution in Chronic Myelogenous Leukemia and Acute Lymphoblastic Leukemia

Because DNA rearrangements serve as unique tumor markers they have enabled us to follow the clonal evolution of individual leukemias over time. This was illustrated within chronic myelogenous leukemia as presented in Figure 6[21]. During acute or chronic granulocytic phases the clonal granulocytes bearing

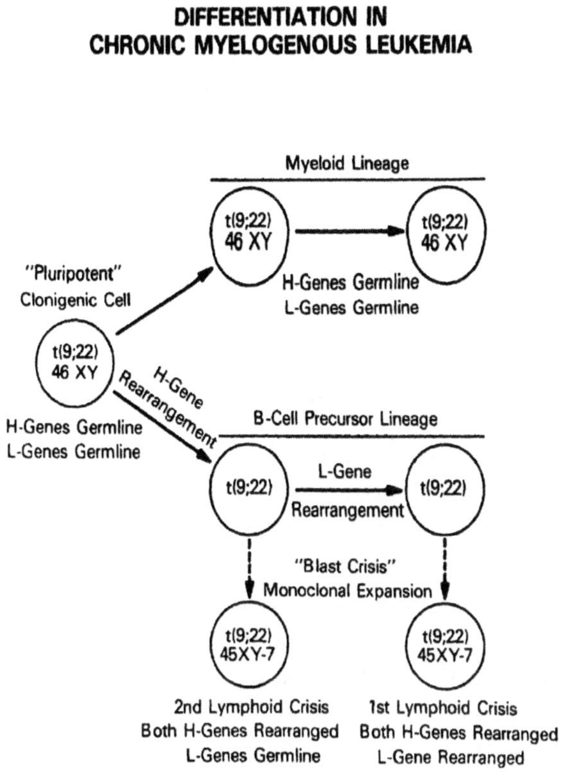

FIGURE 6. The pleuripotent clonigenic cell and myeloid derivation in chronic myelogenous leukemias bear the t(9;22) Philadelphia chromosomal marker and retain germline Ig genes. Two separate lymphoid crises in the same patient have identical H chain gene rearrangements and have lost chromosome 7. However, the first crisis episode had progressed to λ L chain rearrangement whereas the second had germline L chain genes.[21]

the t(9;22) Philadelphia translocation have germline H and L chain genes. Serial examinations of a single patient during clinically distinct episodes of lymphoid blast crisis revealed a differentiation of the affected clone. Both lymphoid crises displayed a new cytogenetic marker consisting of the loss of chromosome 7, 45XY-7 t(9;22) and possessed identical H chain gene rearrangements. However, the two crises could be genetically distinguished[21]. The first lymphoid crisis had progressed to a λ L chain gene rearrangement; whereas, the second lymphoid crisis had germline L chain genes (Fig. 6). Thus, both blast crises shared an ultimate common progenitor cell with doubly rearranged H chain genes. However, the immediate precursor cell which gave rise to each monoclonal expansion varied in their extent of genetic maturation with respect to L chain genes. This indicates that the clonally affected B cell precursors in CML can undergo the sequential differentiative steps of H and L chain rearrangement[21]. Similarly, we have also noted that relapses within pre-B cell ALL can show such normal genetic progression.

Chromosomal Translocations May Also Rearrange the Immunoglobulin Gene Loci

Specific chromosomal translocations are uniquely or highly associated with histologically distinct neoplasms. Curiously, within mature B cell malignancies the sites of chromosomal translocation involve the very bands that contain the Ig genes. In fact, studies of Burkitt lymphomas have revealed that the molecular site of chromosomal breakage can occur within the Ig gene loci themselves (Table 2)[5,6]. In Burkitt lymphoma, the c-myc cellular oncogene locus on chromosome 8 at band q24 is uniformly involved in translocation with the H chain gene at 14q32, κ at 2p11, or λ at 22q11. The introduction of c-myc into a position near an Ig gene locus markedly alters the regulatory control of this gene.

Table 2. Chromosomal translocations in lymphoid neoplasms.

t(8:14) (q24;q32)	Burkitt lymphoma
t(8;22) (q24;q11)	
t(2;8) (p11;q24)	
t(11;14) (q13;q32)	Chronic lymphocytic leukemia
	Small cell lymphocytic lymphoma
	Diffuse large cell lymphoma
t(14;18) (q32;q21)	Follicular small cleaved cell lymphoma
	Follicular mixed cell lymphoma
	Follicular large cell lymphoma
	Diffuse histiocytic lymphoma

As Table 2 indicates, the chromosomal breakpoint of 14q32 repeatedly appears within several other mature B cell neoplasms. A translocation between chromosomes 11q13 and 14q32 is observed in occasional chronic lymphocytic leukemias, small cell lymphocytic lymphomas and diffuse large cell lymphomas. In addition, a remarkably common translocation occurs between 18q21 and 14q32 within the very prevalent follicular and some diffuse lymphomas[24,25]. Thus the H chain gene locus appears to frequently mediate chromosomal translocations in human B cell malignancies. Just as c-myc was rearranged in Burkitt lymphomas, there may well be transformation-related genes located at 11q13 and 18q21. As none of the known c-onc genes map to these locations, these chromosomal translocations may be pivotal in identifying new oncogenes. Croce and his colleagues have used this approach to identify such a candidate gene located at 11q13[26]. Likewise, we have identified a potential oncogene from 18q21. In addition to advancing our understanding of transformation, probes from the sites of these chromosomal breaks detect "malignancy-specific" rearrangements of certain diagnostic utility. Thus chromosomal translocations may serve as an additional form of human gene map. At one site of a chromosomal breakpoint may be a phenotypic landmark gene integral to the counterpart stage of differentiation (e.g., Ig in B cells). The other chromosomal partner may contribute an oncogene which when introduced into its new location has an altered regulation and contributes to the growth or differentiative abnormalities of these tumors.

REFERENCES

1. Aisenberg AC: Cell surface markers in lymphoproliferative disease. N Engl J Med 1978, 304;331-336
2. Rudders RA, Ahl, ET Jr, DeLellis RA: Surface marker and histopathologic correlation with long term survival in advanced large-cell non-Hodgkin's lymphoma. Cancer 1981: 47;1329-35
3. Faguet GB, Webb HH, Agee JF, Ricks WB, Sharbaugh AH: Immunologically diagnosed malignancy in Sjogren's pseudolymphoma. Am J Med 1978; 65;424-429
4. Arnold A, Cossman J, Bakhshi A, Jaffe ES, Waldmann TA and Korsmeyer SJ: Immunoglobulin gene rearrangements as unique clonal markers in human lymphoid neoplasms. N Eng J Med 1983; 309;1593-1599
5. Taub R, Kirsch I, Morton C, Lenoir G, Swan D, Tronick S, Aaronson S, Leder P: Translocation of the c-myc gene into the immunoglobulin heavy chain locus in human Burkitt's lymphoma and murine plasmacytoma cells. Proc Natl Acad Sci USA 1982; 79;7837

6. Nishikura K, Ar-Rushdi A, Erickson J, Watt R, Rovera G, Croce CM: Differential expression of the normal and of the translocated human c-myc oncogenes in B-cells. Proc Natl Acad Sci USA 1983; 80;4822
7. Leder P: The genetics of antibody diversity. Sci Amer 1982; 246;102-115
8. Tonegawa S: Somatic generation of antibody diversity. Nature 1983; 302;575-581
9. Korsmeyer SJ, Hieter PA, Sharrow SO, Goldmann CK, Leder P, and Waldmann TA: Normal human B-cells display ordered light-chain gene rearrangements and deletions. J Exp Med 1982; 156;975-985
10. Cleary MI, Warnke R, and Sklar J: Monoclonality of lymphoproliferative lesions in cardiac transplant recipients. N Engl J Med 1984; 310;477-482
11. Hieter PA, Korsmeyer SJ, Waldmann TA, and Leder P: Human immunoglobulin kappa light chain genes are deleted or rearranged in lambda producing B-cells. Nature 1981; 390;368-372
12. Korsmeyer SJ, Hieter PA, Ravetch JV, Poplack DG, Waldmann and Leder P: A developmental hierarchy of immunoglobulin gene rearrangements in human leukemic pre-B-cells. Proc Natl Acad Sci USA 1981; 78;7096-7100
13. Korsmeyer SJ, Arnold A, Bakhshi A, et al.: Immunoglobulin gene rearrangement and cell surface antigen expression in acute lymphocytic leukemias of T-cell and B-cell precursor origins. J Clin Invest 1983; 71;301-313
14. Nadler LM, Korsmeyer SJ, Anderson KC et al.: The B-cell origin of non-T-cell acute lymphoblastic leukemia: a model for discrete stages of neoplastic and normal pre-B-cell differentiation. J Clin Invest 1984; 74;332-340
15. Nadler LM, Anderson KC, Mouti G, et al.: B_4, a human B-lymphocyte associated antigen expressed on normal, mitogen-activated, and malignant B lymphocytes. J Immunol 1983; 131;244-250
16. Nadler LM, Ritz J, Hardy R, Pesando JM, and Schlossman SF: A unique cell surface antigen identifying lymphoid malignancies of B-cell origin. J Clin Invest 1981; 67;134-141
17. Yanagi Y, Yoshikai Y, Leggett K, Clark SP, Aleksander I and Mak TW; A human T-cell specific cDNA clone encodes a protein having extensive homology to immunoglobulin chains. Nature 1984; 308;145-149
18. Hedrick SM, Cohen DI, Nielson EA and Davis MM: Isolation of cDNA clones encoding T-cell specific membrane-associated proteins. Nature 1984; 308;149-153
19. Chien Y-H, Becker DM, Lindsten T, Okamuras M, Cohen DI, and Davis MM: A third type of murine T-cell receptor gene. Nature 1984; 312;31-35
20. Saito H, Kranz DM, Takagaki Y, Hayday AC, Eisen HN, and Tonegawa S: A third rearranged and expressed gene in a clone of cytotoxic T lymphocytes. Nature 1984; 312;36-40
21. Bakhshi A, Minowada J, Arnold A, Cossman J, Jensen JP, Whang-Peng J, Waldmann TA and Korsmeyer SJ: Lymphoid blast crisis of chronic myelogenous leukemia represent stages in the development of B-cell precursors. New Engl J Med 1983; 309;826-831

22. Ford AM, Molgaard HV, Greaves MF, and Gould HJ: Immunoglobulin gene organization and expression in hematopoietic stem cell leukemia. Embo J 1983; 2;997-1001
23. Korsmeyer SJ, Greene WC, Cossman J et al.: Rearrangement and expression of immunoglobulin genes and expression of Tac antigen in hairy cell leukemia. Proc Natl Acad Sci USA 1983; 80;4522-4526
24. Rowley JD and Testa Jr: Chromosome abnormalities in malignant hematologic diseases. Adv Cancer Res 1982; 36;103-148
25. Yunis JJ: The chromosomal basis of human neoplasia. Science 1983; 221;227-236
26. Tsujimato Y, Yunis J, Onorato-Showe L, Eriksen J, Nowell PC and Croce CM: Molecular cloning of the chromosomal breakpoint of B-cell lymphomas and leukemias with the t(11;14) chromosome translocation. Science 1984; 224;1403-1406

ANIMAL MODELS OF LYMPHOID CELL NEOPLASIA

PAUL PATTENGALE

The goals of this paper are twofold. Firstly, the biologic framework and rationale for the recent redefinition of mouse lymphoid cell neoplasms will be described; and secondly, some recent experiments will be described which document the accelerated development of spontaneous mammary adenocarcinomas in transgenic mice which carry and express MTV/myc fusion genes.

REDEFINITION OF MURINE LYMPHOID CELL NEOPLASMS

Thelma Dunn proposed a classification for mouse hematopoietic cell neoplasms in 1954 which in reality dealt with two major categories of tumors, lymphocytic neoplasms and reticulum cell neoplasms.[1] This designation was principally based on cell size and did not relate to the biologic behavior of these particular neoplasms. In addition, there were categories for plasma cells, and for a so-called undifferentiated group of lymphoid cell neoplasms. This classification persisted until 1981. Since the mouse has excellent experimental accessibility because of its well-defined immunologic system, it appeared logical to redefine mouse lymphoid cell neoplasms. The classification as proposed by Pattengale and Taylor[2-4] is based on both the Lukes/Collins[5] and the Kiel[6] classifications. The goal of this classification was to provide a histopathologic framework for the definition of homogeneous morphologic groups and to further ask whether or not they resembled human disease. Most importantly, these homogeneous morphologic groups could then be amplified and expanded using molecular, cytogenetic and biologic criteria, with an additional major goal being to compare them to the human system.

The proposed classification and its practical usefulness are published elsewhere.[2-4] Briefly, it lists five major morphologic types, which are then combined with immunologic criteria to determine their B or T cell nature (Table 1). In addition to careful

Table 1. Immunomorphologic Classification of Murine Lymphoid Cell Neoplasms as Proposed by Pattengale and Taylor (1981)[1]

Morphologic type[2] (lymphoid cell morphology)	Immunologic type[3] B cell	T cell	Non-B,Non-T cell
Follicular center cell (FCC)[4]			
Small cell type	+	0	0
Large cell type	+	0	0
Large & small (mixed) type	+	0	0
Plasma cell	+	0	0
Immunoblast	+	(+)	(+)
Small lymphocyte	+	(+)	(+)
Lymphoblast	+[5]	+	+

[1]The proposed classification refers only to lymphoid cell, lymphocyte-derived neoplasms and therefore excludes those derived from the monocyte/macrophage/histiocyte series (ie, true histiocytic lymphoma). It is also stressed that the diagnosis of lymphoma/leukemia is based primarily on morphologic criteria and is then subsequently combined with immunologically based parameters.

[2]The morphologic cell types listed are those that have been observed and documented to date. If analogous to man, one would expect to observe additional cell types such as the cerebriform lymphocyte (ie, Sezary-mycosis fungoides T cell) and the plasmacytoid B lymphocyte (ie, Waldenstrom's macroglobulinemia), as well as others.

[3]A B cell is defined as having easily detectable surface and/or cytoplasmic immunoglobulin; a T cell is defined as having easily detectable surface Thy 1 (ie, theta antigen); a non-B non-T cell is defined as lacking both easily detectable Thy-1 and surface and/or cytoplasmic immunoglobulin.

[4]Follicular center cell (FCC) lymphomas with a marked lymph node follicular pattern analogous to those appearing in man have not yet been well documented. FCC lymphomas may also contain equally prominent mixtures of both large and small FCC type (FCC lymphoma--mixed--large and small cell types).

[5]Lymphoblastic lymphoma of B cells is considered by some to be an FCC lymphoma and by others to be a separate category. In either event, it closely resembles the Burkitt's lymphoma spectrum.

+ = already observed and documented
(+) = not yet observed, but expected
0 = not observed nor expected

phenotyping, it should be emphasized that the designation of T or B cell nature can now be made at the genomic DNA level as measured by gene rearrangement of either T or B cell antigen receptors. I also want to stress that the follicular center cell (FCC) morphologic types as originally defined by Lukes/Collins and Lennert are highly predictive of a B cell nature. This is, of course, also true of the plasma cell category. Table 2 compares the Dunn classification[1] to the Pattengale/Taylor classification.[2]

Lymphomas are lymphoid cell neoplasms, and by definition, are malignant. Clinically speaking, some morphologic types are predictably high grade, while others are intermediate or low-grade malignancies. The pathologist is therefore trying to make a morphologic assessment which will be predictive of clinical behavior and will therefore be helpful to the clinician. An additional important point is that low-grade lymphomas, such as small FCC lymphomas, can progress with time to intermediate grades (eg, mixed FCC) and to high grades (eg, large FCC). A classification should therefore be clinically useful. In addition, a classification should also be scientifically accurate, easily taught, easily learned, and reproducible.

The scientific accuracy of a neoplastic lymphoid cell classification has also allowed us to make definitive statements about lymphoid cell differentiation, particularly with regard to B cells. If one believes that lymphomas are arrests in the differentiation pathway, one can obtain reasonably homogeneous populations of B cell types at various stages of differentiation. Lymphomas or lymphoid cell neoplasms have therefore been powerful tools in understanding the immunobiology of normal B cells.

Lymphoid progenitor cells can go to either the B or T cell arm, depending on how the cell wants to rearrange its DNA. If it goes to the B cell side through the pre-B series, it will rearrange its immunoglobulin genes (heavy mu followed by kappa followed by lambda) and express mu heavy chain in its cytoplasm. The earliest B cell which has easily detectable surface immunoglobulin is an early or immature B cell which has surface IgM associated with one or the other light chains. These lymphomas of early B cells, which are called by some,[2-4,6] "B cell lymphoblastic lymphomas," and by others,[5] "small non-cleaved follicular cell lymphomas," are the Burkitt's lymphoma types. One can also observe lymphoblastic

Table 2. Comparison of the Classifications for Murine Lymphoma and Related Leukemias[1]

Dunn (1954)	Pattengale/Taylor (1981)
	Lymphoblastic lymphoma
Lymphocytic neoplasm	Small lymphocytic lymphoma
	FCC lymphoma--small cell
RCN Type A[2] -----------	FCC lymphoma--large cell
	FCC lymphoma--large & small cell (mixed)
RCN Type B[3]	Immunoblastic lymphoma
Plasma cell[4] neoplasm	Plasma cell lymphoma

[1]As proposed by Dunn, lymphocytic neoplasms can be localized (ie, lymphoma) or generalized (ie, leukemia) involving the peripheral blood and bone marrow compartments. By comparison and direct analogy, lymphomas of lymphoblasts, small lymphocytes, and follicular center cells can manifest with leukemic phases (ie, lymphoma/-leukemias). RCN, Type C is considered by Dunn to be nonneoplastic and nonlymphoid in origin.

[2]Most RCNs (reticulum cell neoplasms) Type A, as proposed by Dunn, are considered to be derived from true histiocytic cells (ie, true nonlymphoid, phagocytic histiocytes) and rarely can present as a monocytic leukemia. The dotted line stresses the fact that a few tumors morphologically classified as RCN, Type A may represent large FCC lymphomas.

[3]Although RCN, Type B is now considered NOT to be representative of Hodgkin's disease, it can include both prelymphomatous, nonneoplastic lymphoproliferations and true lymphoid cell lymphomas (mixed FCC and immunoblastic cell types). A lymphoma is defined as a lymphoid cell neoplasm (ie, an autonomous monoclonal new growth, presumably derived from one cell). In contrast, a prelymphoma is defined as a conditioned, atypical lymphoid cell hyperplasia derived from more than one cell (nonmonoclonal, oligoclonal, or polyclonal derivation), with a propensity to progress to a true lymphoid cell neoplasm with time.

[4]As stated by Dunn, a proportion of plasma cell neoplasms were formed by typical well-differentiated plasma cells, while others were formed of a cell type resembling a reticulum cell (ie, a B immunoblast with plasmacytoid features). This concept was in agreement with the Rask-Nielsen classification of plasma cell neoplasms. It should be noted that the term "plasma cell leukemia" was used to denote a localized growth (lymphoma). True plasma cell leukemia with peripheral blood and bone marrow involvement is rare.

morphology in the pre-B series. Mature, virgin B cells have the morphology of resting small lymphocytes. Lymphomas of small lymphocytes (CLL cells), similar to mature, virgin B cells co-express surface IgM and IgD. Follicular center cell (FCC) lymphomas are farther along in B cell differentiation and most often have class-switched to other immunoglobulin classes (usually IgG and IgA), which can now be easily detected in the cytoplasm. Lymphomas of B immunoblasts and plasma cells are characterized as post-follicular B cells, which are closer to terminal differentiation and are actively secreting immunoglobulin.

Clearly, these B cell neoplasms have resulted in a more precise definition of morphologic B cell subtypes which has direct application to B cell differentiation. This has also been applied to frozen section methodology using monoclonal antibodies, which relates precise phenotypic characterization to intact histopathologic microanatomy.

When this classification was proposed by Pattengale and Taylor,[2-4] enough case material was then accumulated in the mouse, which enabled us to make a definitive statement as to whether or not the mouse does resemble the human with regard to lymphoid cell neoplasms. Table 3 demonstrates that in 383 spontaneous lymphoid cell neoplasms occurring in aged inbred strains, the vast majority were found to be B cell-derived, follicular center cell (FCC) types. This is remarkably similar to the age-related incidence of FCC types as seen in adult human non-Hodgkin's lymphoma.[7-8] Also as observed in the human, smaller numbers of immunoblastic, lymphoblastic and small lymphocytic types have been documented. It can now be said with some confidence that in both mouse and man, B cell lymphomas are much more common than T cell lymphomas, especially if one looks at the spontaneous incidence in aged mice. It again should be stressed that the murine system is well-defined, both genetically and immunologically, and is experimentally accessible for carefully controlled, prospective studies. If you have such a well-defined animal system, and it bears some resemblance to human disease, one can now use this animal (eg, murine) system to obtain experimental information that you could not otherwise get from the human system.

As previously stated, an important approach to lymphoid cell neoplasms in the mouse is to further define homogeneous,

Table 3. Immunomorphologic Classification of 383 Spontaneous Murine Lymphoid Cell Neoplasms[1]

# cases	Morphologic Diagnosis	# of CIg+[2] / # Tested[3]	%CIg+
279	Follicular center cell (FCC)[4]	168/200	84
45	Immunoblast	28/32	88
4	Plasma cell	4/4	100
35	Lymphoblast	12/20	60
20	Small lymphocyte	nt[5]	nt[5]
383	TOTAL	212/256[3]	83

[1]Includes 70 BALB/C, 111 $B6C3F_1$s, 62 NFS/N (V-congeneics), 69 $B6CBAF_1$s, 30 C57BL/6, and 41 mice from miscellaneous inbred strains. With the exception of the NFS/N, V-congeneics, which develop spontaneous lymphomas at approximately 12-18 months of age, the vast majority (>95%) of the remaining strains were greater than 18 months of age.

[2]Positivity for CIg is determined by the presence of easily detectable cytoplasmic immunoglobulin in greater than 25% of the critical neoplastic cells using conventional immunoperoxidase staining on fixed, paraffin-embedded tissues.

[3]Not all cases were tested (ie, 127 of 383) primarily due to inadequate fixation of lymphoid tissues.

[4]Of the 279 FCC lymphomas, 147 were large FCC type, 97 were mixed FCC type, and 35 were small FCC type.

[5]nt=not tested. Due to the scant amount of cytoplasm in the small lymphocytic type, cytoplasmic immunoglobulin cannot be properly evaluated.

experimentally accessible, immunobiologic subgroups at the cytogenetic and molecular level. For example, when one examines the genomic DNA of a spontaneous lymphoblastic lymphoma of B cells and compares it to non-Burkitt B cell types such as FCC, immunoblastic and small lymphocytic lymphomas, it was found that this Burkitt equivalent in the mouse had a structurally rearranged 3.6kb c-myc fragment which was not present in the other lymphoma types (Figure 1).

In summary, mouse lymphoid cell neoplasms are excellent models for human disease.

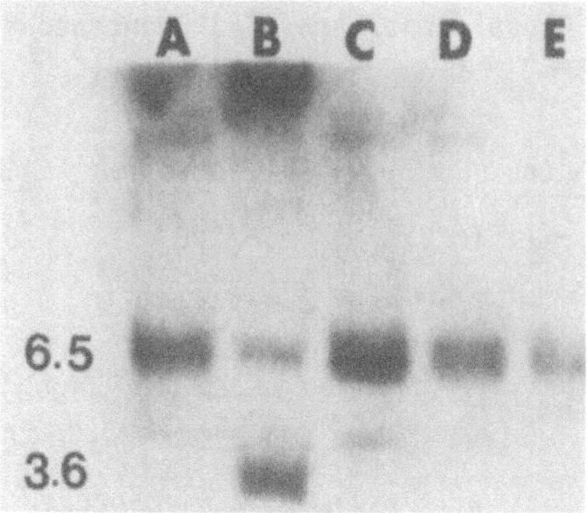

FIGURE 1. EcoR1 digest and Southern blot of genomic DNA from lymphoma cells occurring spontaneously in NFS/N, V-congeneic mice. Hybridization with ^{32}P nick-translated v-myc probe performed under low stringency conditions. Please note the rearranged 3.6 kb c-myc fragment in Lane B as compared to Lanes A,C,D,E.

Lane A: normal spleen
Lane B: lymphoblastic lymphoma of B cells (spleen)
Lane C: immunoblastic lymphoma of B cells (spleen)
Lane D: small lymphocytic lymphoma of B cells (spleen)
Lane E: large FCC lymphoma of B cells (spleen)

ACCELERATED DEVELOPMENT OF SPONTANEOUS MAMMARY ADENOCARCINOMAS IN TRANSGENEIC MICE CARRYING AND EXPRESSING MTV/myc FUSION GENES

These experiments are described in more detail in a separate publication.[9] Briefly, MTV/myc fusion genes of various constructions were injected into the male pronuclei of fertilized C57BL/6 females which had been impregnated with CD-1 sperm. CD-1 is an outbred strain of mice, in contrast to C57BL/6 which is an inbred strain. Thirteen founder strains were generated which carried a particular type of MTV/myc construct, which had been placed in the germ line DNA of single cell embryos. The fusion genes consisted of a normal mouse c-myc gene in which increasingly larger portions of the myc promoter region were replaced by the hormonally inducible mouse mammary tumor virus (MTV) promoter. The hormone inducibility of the MTV promotor involves its interaction with glucocorticoids. These contructions are described in detail elsewhere.[9]

At four to seven months of age, the female founders of two of these transgenic strains spontaneously developed mammary adenocarcinomas during one of their early pregnancies (Figure 2).

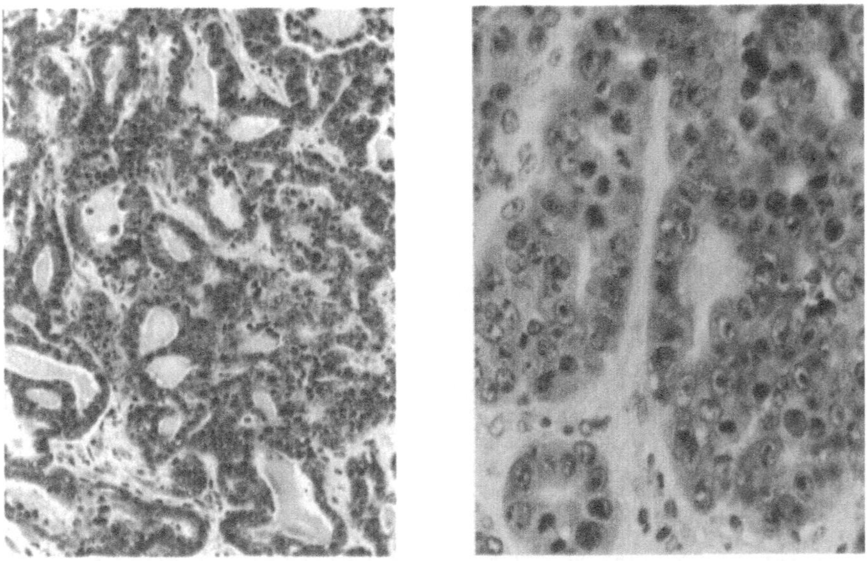

(A) (B)

FIGURE 2. Histologic appearance of spontaneous mammary tumor occurring in founder mouse 141-3. (A) Low-power view of malignant mammary adenocarcinoma demonstrating moderate differentiation (subcutaneous mammary tissue, 320x, hematoxylin and eosin); (B) High-power view of primary mammary tumor demonstrating malignant epithelial glands (subcutaneous mammary tissue, 640x, hematoxylin and eosin).

Interestingly, both the mammary tumors, as well as the residual non-neoplastic breast tissue, expressed RNA transcripts corresponding to the fusion genes. It should be stressed that C57BL/6 and CD-1 mice have a very low incidence of spontaneous mammary adenocarcinoma which only occurs in old age.

In the best studied founder strain, designated as 141-3, spontaneous mammary adenocarcinomas were observed in all the available female progeny, which had inherited the same gene, and which were in their first or second pregnancies.

In summary, it should be stressed that spontaneous lymphoid cell neoplasms in the mouse bear a close resemblance to human lymphoid cell neoplasms. One can now proceed in the mouse system with relevant molecular and cytogenetic questions. It should also be stressed that transgenic mice have been useful in generating a Mendelian inheritance pattern for certain types of neoplasms, particularly adenocarcinomas and more recently lymphomas (Aya and

Philip Leder, personal communication). In the next five to ten years, the mouse will probably provide us with the mechanistic understanding for the development of malignant neoplasms.

REFERENCES

1. Dunn TB. 1954. Normal and pathologic anatomy of the reticular tissue in laboratory mice, with a classification and discussion of neoplasms. J Natl Cancer Inst 14:1281-1433.
2. Pattengale PK, Taylor P, Twomey P, Hill S, Jonasson J, Beardsley T, Haas M. 1982. Immunopathology of B cell lymphomas induced in C57BL/6 mice by dualtropic murine leukemia virus (MuLV). Am J Pathol 107:362-377.
3. Pattengale PK, Frith CH. 1983. Immunomorphologic classification of spontaneous lymphoid cell neoplasms occurring in female BALB/c mice. J Natl Cancer Inst 70:169-179.
4. Pattengale PK, Taylor CR. 1983. Experimental models of lymphoproliferative disease: the mouse as a model for human non-Hodgkin's lymphomas and related leukemias. Am J Pathol 113:237-265.
5. Lukes RJ, Collins RD. 1975. New approaches to the classification of the lymphomata. Br J Cancer 31 (Suppl 2):1-28.
6. Lennert K, Stein H, Kaiserling E. 1975. Cytological and functional criteria for the classification of malignant lymphomata. Br J Cancer 31 (suppl 2):29-43.
7. Lukes RJ, Taylor CR, Parker JW, Lincoln TL, Pattengale PK, Tindle BH. 1978. Morphological and immunologic surface marker study of 299 cases of non-Hodgkin's lymphomas and related leukemias. Am J Pathol 90:461-485.
8. Lukes RJ, Taylor CR, Parker JW. 1982. Immunologic surface marker studies in the histopathological diagnosis of non-Hodgkin's lymphomas based on multiparameter studies of 790 cases. In: Advances in Malignant Lymphoma: Etiology, Immunology, Pathology, and Treatment, Vol 3. Rosenberg SA, Kaplan HS (eds). New York, Academic Press.
9. Stewart TA, Pattengale PK, Leder P. 1984. Spontaneous mammary adenocarcinomas in transgenic mice that carry and express MTV/myc fusion genes. Cell 38:627-637.

A NEW LOOK AT THE RELATIONSHIP OF THE IMMUNE SYSTEM TO NEOPLASIA

GUNTHER DENNERT

INTRODUCTION

The participation of specific immune effectors in the surveillance and controls of spontaneously arising neoplasia has been an important hypothesis for many years. The unique appeal of this hypothesis to cellular immunologists came from the observation of continuous and systematic rejection of altered body cells by cytotoxic T lymphocytes. Soon apparent, however, was the disconcerting observation that congenitally immunodeficient athymic nude mice, which lack functional T cells, had no greater incidence of primary spontaneous, virally or chemically induced neoplasia than normal mice.[1] It is in this context that the discovery of natural killer (NK) cells, which are present in both normal and thymus-deficient mice, renewed hopes that immunological surveillance of neoplasia might be a real phenomenon.[2] Natural killer cells are a minor population of lymphoid cells that are capable of lysing a variety of transformed cells and virus-infected cells apparently without requiring prior exposure to antigens.[3] Recently it was discovered that NK cells can be activated by interferons and also by interleukin 2, leading to the establishment of in vitro cell clones[4,5] that could be used to directly test the hypothesis that NK cells play a role in the immunosurveillance of neoplasia.[6] The following is a discussion of current knowledge and evidence for this hypothesis.

EVIDENCE FOR AN IN VITRO FUNCTION OF NK CELLS: THE BONE MARROW REJECTION MODEL

For NK cells to achieve credibility beyond their cytotoxic effect in vitro, it had to be shown that they perform some important function in vivo. Many years ago the late Gustavo Cudkovicz and collaborators found a genetic association between NK activity and the acute rejection of allogenic bone marrow grafts.[7] The antigen on the bone marrow graft that was recognized was coded closely to the H-2D region and was called Hh (hemopoietic histocompatibility) antigen. This observation gave rise to the notion that NK cells may be important not only for acute rejection of marrow grafts, but also for the surveillance of bone marrow growth and differentiation.

Genetically NK-deficient beige mice,[8] or mice made selectively NK deficient by irradiation,[9] fail to acutely reject allogenic bone marrow grafts. This defect can be restored by reconstituting, for instance, beige mice with the cloned NK cell line NKB61A2 (Table 1). Since marrow graft rejection shows exquisite specificity for the Hh antigens encoded close to H-2D, it is important to ascertain that graft rejection subsequent to NK clone injection into NK-deficient mice shows the same specificity. In Table 2 it is seen that C57BL/6 mice ($H\text{-}2^b$) heterozygous for the bg mutation (bg/+) show specific rejection of ($H\text{-}2^d$) marrow grafts which maps primarily to H-2D, while mice that carry the homozygous bg mutation do not reject $H\text{-}2^d$ marrow grafts. Injection of NKB61B10 into homozygous beige mice results in a specific rejection of the $H\text{-}2^d$ marrow graft, which again shows specificity for the H-2D region of the major histocompatibility gene complex (MHC). This result clearly showed that NK-mediated marrow graft rejection can be $H\text{-}2D^d$ specific. But it also raised the important question how NK cells, which, from all that is known from in vitro cytotoxicity assays, are not capable of recognizing H-2 antigens, acquire this specificity in vivo. Recent experiments by us have shown that the putative H-2 specificity of NK cells in marrow graft rejection is very likely due to preexisting natural anti-H-2 antibody in the marrow graft recipient. Consequently, serum of the C57BL/6 ($H\text{-}2^b$) mouse, which is capable of rejecting a Balb/C ($H\text{-}2^d$) marrow graft is able to transfer the ability to reject a Balb/C ($H\text{-}2^d$) marrow graft to strain 129/SvJ recipient mice (Table 3). Again it can be shown that the specificity of rejection maps to the H-2D region, as is the case in the C57BL/6 mouse.

These results point to two important conclusions: NK cells are able to cause marrow graft rejection, and this rejection involves the participation of humoral antibody which serves as an NK receptor. NK cells may therefore attach to their targets in two ways. In one, their own receptor is used, i.e., the one that is usually assayed in vitro in the absence of antibody. In the other, anti-

Table 1

MARROW REJECTION: REQUIREMENT FOR CELLS WITH NK ACTIVITY

Irradiated recipient given BALB/c marrow	Cell lines+ injected on day-7 (NK activity)	Splenic ^{125}IUdR uptake (%)
C57BL/6	none	1 ± 1
C57BL/6 bg	none	100 ± 12
C57BL/6 bg	NKB61A2 (+)	2 ± 1
C57BL/6 bg	CTLL-2 (-)	97 ± 19
C57BL/6 bg	BB1 (-)	87 ± 25
BALB/c	none	82 ± 21

+All cell lines require Con A CM for continuous growth.

Table 2

Genetic Specificity of NK-Mediated Bone Marrow Allograft Rejection

Donor Bone Marrow			
Strain	H-2 KISD	Irradiated* C57BL/6 (H-2^b) Recipient	Donor Bone+ Marrow Growth
B10	b b b b	bg/+	100 ± 10
B10.D2	d d d d	bg/+	1 ± 1
B10.A (18R)	b b b d	bg/+	8 ± 2
D2.GD	d d b b	bg/+	30 ± 3
B10	b b b b	bg/bg	68 ± 10
B10.D2	d d d d	bg/bg	70 ± 5
B10.A (18R)	b b b d	bg/bg	64 ± 3
D2.GD	d d b b	bg/bg	90 ± 12
B10	b b b b	bg/bg + NK**	70 ± 8
B10.D2	d d d d	bg/bg + NK	2 ± 1
B10.A (18R)	b b b d	bg/bg + NK	6 ± 1
D2.GD	d d b b	bg/bg + NK	26 ± 2

*Lethally irradiated recipients were injected with 1 x 10^6 donor bone marrow cells.

**Injected with 2 x 10^6 cloned NK cells (NKB61B10) four days before transplantation.

+Values relative to syngeneic growth controls arbitrarily set at 100 units.

Table 3

Genetic Specificity of Bone Marrow Graft Rejection Following Transfer of Serum from Responder Mice

Donor Bone Marrow Strain	H-2 K I S D	Irradiated* $H-2^b$ Recipient	Donor Bone+ Marrow Growth
A. B10	b b b b	C57BL/6	90 ± 4
B10.D2	d d d d	C57BL/6	7 ± 2
B10.A (18R)	b b b d	C57BL/6	13 ± 3
D2.GD	d d b b	C57BL/6	82 ± 10
B. B10	b b b b	129/SvJ	100 ± 13
B10.D2	d d d d	129/SvJ	100 ± 4
B10.A (18R)	b b b d	129/SvJ	98 ± 10
D2.GD	d d b b	129/SvJ	100 ± 15
C. B10	b b b b	129/SvJ + C57BL/6 serum**	120 ± 18
B10.D2	d d d d	129/SvJ + C57BL/6 serum	9 ± 3
B10.A (18R)	b b b d	129/SvJ + C57BL/6 serum	18 ± 2
D2.GD	d d b b	129/SvJ + C57BL/6 serum	91 ± 15

*Lethally irradiated recipients were transplanted with 1×10^6 donor bone marrow cells and marrow growth assayed 6 days later. Values relative to syngeneic growth control of 100 units.

**Irradiated recipient mice were injected with a mixture of donor bone marrow and serum (1:4) collected from C57BL/6 mice.

target cell antibody induces the NK cell to lyse its target in an antibody-dependent cell-mediated cytotoxic reaction (ADCC).

DO NK-DEFICIENT ANIMALS HAVE A HIGH INCIDENCE OF SPONTANEOUS OR INDUCED TUMORS?

The observation that NK cells play an important part in the rejection of marrow grafts sets the stage for the next question, i.e., whether NK cells play a similarly important role in the surveillance of neoplasia. Clearly if this were the case NK-deficient animals should have a high incidence of tumors. While this has not been demonstrated in the case of NK-deficient mice, in humans with the Chediak Higashi Syndrome, also resulting in NK deficiency, there seems to be a prevalence of lymphoproliferative disorders that may be due to neoplastic transformation.[10] It is important to note that the degree of NK deficiency in the Chediak

Higashi Syndrome in humans is more severe than in the beige mouse. Hence, the failure to demonstrate high tumor insistance in beige mice may be due to the presence of residual NK activity in these mice.

In order to obtain further evidence for the participation of NK cells in tumor surveillance, use was made of the observation that irradiation of four week old C57BL/6 mice with four weekly doses of irradiation results in severe suppression of NK activity and the subsequent appearance of and death from thymic leukemia.[9,11] If NK cells indeed play a role in the protection from radiation-induced leukemia, then reconstitution of irradiated mice with NK cells should result in protection from leukemia. Results in Table 4 show that this is indeed the case. Injection of irradiated mice with one dose of NK clone NKB61A2 early after the last irradiation results in a dramatic suppression of death from leukemia. Furthermore, the mice dying from leukemia, although they received NK cells, did so at a significantly later time. It is also important to note that late injections of NK cells had little protective effect, and that injection of CTTL-2 failed to show any protection. These results show that NK cells may have a protective effect in radiation-induced thymic leukemia, but do not answer the still open question whether animals with no NK activity whatsoever would have a higher incidence of spontaneous neoplasia.

Table 4

SUPPRESSION OF IRRADIATION-INDUCED THYMIC LEUKEMIA IN C57BL/6 MICE INJECTED WITH CLONED NK CELLS

Injected cell line[+]	Time (weeks) of injection	Incidence of thymic leukemia (12 months)	Mean appearance time of leukemia (weeks ± S.E.)
none	none	85%	24.2 ± 1.9
NKB61A2	0	20%	42.3 ± 4.9
NKB61A2	4	40%	27.6 ± 3.2
NKB61A2	8	50%	21.4 ± 2.9
NKB61A2	12	80%	24.9 ± 3.3
CTLL-2	0	90%	21.3 ± 2.5

[+]Mice received 4 weekly-doses of 200 rads γ-irradiation. Groups of mice (10-12) received a single injection of $2x10^6$ indicated cells following last irradiation.

NK CELLS HAVE A PROTECTIVE EFFECT AGAINST TRANSPLANTABLE TUMORS AND VIRAL INFECTIONS.

A classical way to examine whether tumors are susceptible to immune attack has been transplantation of such tumors into immuno-deficient mice. Using this approach, it had been shown that the C57BL/6 melanoma B16 forms more experimental metastases in NK-deficient beige mice than in normal mice.[12-14] Therefore, if NK cells indeed control the spread of this tumor, then injection of cloned NK cells should inhibit it. In Table 5, it is seen that tumor-injected NK-deficient mice, in contrast to tumor-injected normal mice, develop increased numbers of pulmonary metastases three weeks after injection. Injection of NKB61A2 at the time of tumor challenge results in a dramatic suppression of tumor metastases. There was, however, little effect when the NK cells were injected at later times, nor was there any effect of a cell line not expressing NK activity (CTLL-2). These results show that NK cells are particularly effective as a first bullwark of defense, but have little effect on established progressively growing tumors.

Table 5

SUPPRESSION OF LUNG TUMOR FORMATION IN NK-DEFICIENT MICE INJECTED WITH NK CELLS AND B16 MELANOMA

Recipient+	Injected cells (NK activity)	Day of Injection	Lung tumor colonies mean ± S.D.
C57BL/6	none	none	37 ± 7
C57BL/6 bg	none	none	139 ± 25
C57BL/6 bg	NKB61A2 (+)	0	43 ± 28
C57BL/6 bg	CTLL-2 (-)	0	131 ± 11
C57BL/6 bg	none	none	267 ± 12
C57BL/6 bg	NKB61A2 (+)	0	83 ± 10
C57BL/6 bg	NKB61A2 (+)	4	118 ± 35
C57BL/6 bg	NKB61A2 (+)	8	159 ± 13
C57BL/6 bg	NKB61A2 (+)	12	193 ± 13
C57BL/6 bg	CTLL-2 (-)	0	260 ± 25

+Mice were injected i.v. with B16 melanoma tumor cells ($1x10^5$) on day 0 and with cloned cells ($2x10^6$) on the indicated days.

Perhaps the most dramatic effect of NK cells as a primary protective mechanism in experimental animals has been achieved with the murine cytomegalovirus (MCMV). It had been shown that the resistance of mice to MCMV infection correlates with their NK activity[15,16] and that newborn mice that are low in NK activity are highly sensitive to MCMV. In a recent study,[17] suckling mice were injected with NK cell clone NKB61B10 in adoptive transfer experiments and subsequently infected with MCMV. Results showed that NK clone injection reduced the MCMV titers about 500 fold. Moreover, 75% of the mice receiving cloned NK cells survived, compared to 0% of the control mice. Similar, but not quite as dramatic effects, can be seen in NK-deficient adult mice. These results confirm that NK cells may indeed play an important part in the primary defense, not only against several transplantable tumors, like the B16 melanoma, but also against several viral infections. It is important to note, however, that there are many tumor and viral systems in which NK cells do not appear to play a protective role. Lymphocytic choriomeningitis (LCM) virus production, for instance, is not influenced by the presence of NK cells.[17]

CAN NK CELLS BE USEFUL IN THE TREATMENT OF PROGRESSIVELY GROWING TUMORS?

The results so far presented show that NK cells have a protective role against radiation-induced leukemia, a transplantable melanoma and viral infection with MCMV. In these experiments, it was important that the NK cells were present at the time of tumor induction or transplantation. Once tumors were progressively growing, there was little protective effect of the NK cells. This suggests that NK cells have a primary protective role, but may have little or no effect once the tumor is progressively growing. In order for NK cells to play a practical role in clinical oncology, it would be important if they could be induced to also eliminate tumor cells in progressively growing neoplasia. To discuss this possibility we have to consider the mechanisms by which NK cells recognize their targets. From in vitro experiments it is clear that NK cells attach to and lyse a selected number of tumor cells, and presently it is not clear what antigens are recognized on these lysable NK targets. It is also known that NK cells cause specific bone marrow graft rejection, and there is strong evidence that this rejection mechanism involves the participation of serum antibody present in the graft recipient. Moreover, it is well known that NK cells are able to lyse targets in an antibody-dependent cytolytic reaction (ADCC). One way to enhance the effectivity of NK cell lysis, therefore, would be to provide them with specific antitarget cell antibody.

In a recent publication, Schulz, Bumol and Reisfeld[18] reported that a monoclonal antibody 9.2.27 specific for the human melanoma M21 induces tumor suppression in nude mice. It was suspected that this effect was due to antibody-directed NK-like effectors, and we therefore decided to analyze this phenomenon with the aim to explore whether NK cells may indeed be able to cause rejection of progressively growing tumors if and when specific antibody was given to aid NK cytolysis. First, it was important to ascertain that M21 tumor growth in nude mice is indeed subject to NK inhibition. Nude mice were injected with antiasialo GM1 serum prior to tumor transplantation to eliminate NK cells. Results showed[19] that in such NK-deficient mice the tumor take increased from 20% in untreated nude mice to 100% in antiasiolo GM1-treated mice and that the tumor volume was 2-3 times larger in the antiasialo GM1-treated NK-deficient mice. This result showed that M21 tumor growth in nude mice is indeed subject to suppression by NK cells. The next question then was whether progressively growing tumors could be influenced by injection of NK cells and antibody specific for the melanoma. Results showed that injection of antibody only into tumor-bearing mice has little effect, but injection of both antibody and cell populations with NK activity resulted in a 70% tumor regression and about tenfold suppression of tumor volume in those mice in which the tumor did not regress. The dramatic effect was apparently due to cells with NK activity, since normal splenocytes and spenocytes from nude mice injected with the antibody into tumor-bearing mice caused the effect. In contrast, splenocytes from NK-deficient beige mice could not be shown to have aany effects, whereas injection of tumor-bearing mice with antibody and a cloned NK cell line again showed tumor suppression. These results strongly suggest that NK cells may, under certain conditions, cause tumor regression if they are also supplied with a specific antitumor antibody.

CONCLUSIONS

Our studies with cloned cell lines expressing NK activity have provided compelling evidence for the role of NK cells in acute bone marrow graft rejection. The results have also formed the basis for the hypothesis that NK cells may play a regulatory role in the development of hemopoeitic stem cells and/or their progeny. While this hypothesis is quite speculative presently, it seems now well proven that NK cells play an important role in protection from certain viral infections and tumors. The function of NK cells in these systems is that of a primary defense mechanism against an invading infection or arising neoplastic cell, which is precisely what one would expect from an effective immunosurveillance mechanism. Our studies in the bone marrow rejection system pointed to the importance of humoral antibody in NK-mediated target cell obstruction. On the other hand, in vitro cytotoxicity studies with NK cells pointed to an antibody independent cytotoxic mechanism that only relies on the specificity of the NK antigen receptor. We have concluded from these two observations that NK-mediated cytolysis may proceed via these two mechanisms in vivo and in vitro. Immunosurveillance by NK cells, therefore, would be expected to similarly progress via two pathways, namely, one which is antibody independent, and the other which is dependent on naturally present antibody. The lack of immunosurveillance against certain tumors, therefore, may be due to either a lack of recognition by NK receptors, the absence of specific antibody or both. It is clear that such a deficiency may be correctable by supplying antibody of appropriate specificity, and recent hybridoma technology provides a very powerful tool in this respect. A demonstration of this approach is the finding that a human melanoma progressively growing in mice may be induced to regress after injection of a tumor-specific antibody and NK effector cells. This, of course, provides us with a potentially important clinical approach to the treatment of metastases of certain tumors in humans. The next years will show whether the rapidly developing field of natural cytotoxicity will bear the fruits promised by these experiments.

REFERENCES

1. Outzen HC, Custer RP, Eaton GJ, Prehn RT. 1975. Spontaneous and induced tumor incidence in germ free nude mice. Res J Reticuloendothel Soc 17:1.
2. Haller O, Hansson M, Kiessling R, Wigzell H. 1977. Role of nonconventional natural killer cells in resistance against syngeneic cells in vivo. Nature 270:609.
3. Herberman RB, Holden HT. 1978. Natural cell mediated immunity. Adv Cancer Res 27:305.
4. Dennert G. 1980. Cloned cell lines of natural killer cells. Nature 287:47.
5. Dennert G, Yogeeswaran G, Yamagata S. 1981. Cloned cell lines with natural killer activity. Specificity, function and cell surface markers. J Exp Med 153:545.
6. Warner JF, Dennert G. 1982. Effect of a cloned cell line with NK activity on bone marrow transplants, tumor development and metastasis. Nature 300:31.
7. Kiessling R, Hochman PS, Shearer GM, Wigzell H, Cudkowicz G. 1977. Evidence for a similar or common mechanism for natural killer cell activity and resistance to hemopoietic grafts. Eur J Immunol 7:655.
8. Roder JC, Duwe AK. The beige mutation in the mouse selectively impairs natural killer cell function. Nature 278:451.
9. Parkinson DR, Brightman RP, Waksal SD. 1981. Altered natural killer cell biology in C57Bl/6 mice after leukemogenic split dose irradiation. J Immunol 126:1460.
10. Dent PB, Fish JF, White, Good RA. 1966. Chediak-Higashi Syndrome: observations on the nature of the associated malignancy. Lab Invest 15:1634.
11. Kaplan HS, Brown MB. 1952. A quantitative dose response study of lymphoid tumor development in irradiated C57Bl/6 mice. J Natl Cancer Inst 13:185.
12. Hanna N, Fidler J. 1980. Role of natural killer cells in the destruction of circulating tumor emboli. J Natl Cancer Inst 65:801.
13. Talmadge JE, Meyers KM, Prieur DJ, Starkey JR. 1980. Role of NK cells in tumor growth and metastasis in beige mice. Nature 284:622.
14. Hanna N, Burton RC. 1981. Definitive evidence that natural killer cells inhibit experimental tumor metastasis in vivo. J Immunol 127:1754.
15. Bancroft GJ, Shellam GR, Chalmer JE. 1981. Genetic influences on the augmentation of natural killer cells during murine cytomegalovirus infection: correlation with patterns of resistance. J Immunol 126:988.
16. Shellam GR, Allen JE, Papadimitoiou JM, Bancroft GJ. 1981. Increased susceptibility to cytomegalovirus infection in beige mutant mice. Proc Natl Acad Sci 78:5104.
17. Bukowski JF, Warner JF, Dennert G, Welsh R. 1985 (in press). Adoptive transfer studies demonstrating the antiviral effects of natural killer cells in vivo. J Exp Med.
18. Schulz G, Bumol TF, Reisfeld RA. 1983. Monoclonal antibody directed effector cells selectively lyse human melanoma cells in vitro and in vivo. Proc Natl Acad Sci USA 80:5407.
19. Schulz G, Staffileno L, Reisfeld RA, Dennert G. 1985 (submitted). Eradication of established human melanoma tumors by antibody directed effector cells with NK activity.

THE EPIDEMIOLOGY OF LYMPHOMAS

RONALD K. ROSS, RUTH L. DWORSKY, ANNLIA PAGANINI-HILL,
PETER NICHOLS

HODGKIN'S DISEASE

Hodgkin's Disease (HD) is relatively well studied epidemiologically. Although a clear understanding of the etiology remains elusive, the descriptive epidemiology of HD has been useful in developing hypotheses regarding etiology.

In Los Angeles, the data for descriptive epidemiologic studies comes from the Cancer Surveillance Program, a population-based tumor registry established in 1970. This program attempts the early identification of all newly diagnosed cancer cases among the nearly 8 million residents of Los Angeles County. Since 1972, over 95% of Los Angeles County incident cancer cases have been registered by this program.

The major conclusion from the descriptive epidemiology of HD in Los Angeles is that it may be two distinct diseases; the nodular sclerosis (NS) subtype has demographic characteristics which are distinct from the other histologic types (1). For example, unlike the non-NS subtypes, NS HD occurs with equal frequency among men and women (Table 1), and with increasing frequency with increasing social class (Table 2). It is the only subtype for which Mexican-Americans show a deficit in incidence compared to other whites. Moreover, NS HD is the only histologic type with a distinct young adult peak, present in both men and women.

Table 1. Average Annual Incidence Rate of Hodgkin's Disease by Race, Sex, and Histology in Los Angeles *

Histology	White Males	White Females	Black All	Mexican-American All
Nodular sclerosis (NS)	1.04	1.00	0.59	0.43
Mixed cellularity (MS)	1.13	0.58	0.73	0.79
Lymphocyte predominance (LP)	0.44	0.26	0.16	0.27
Lymphocyte depletion (LD)	0.39	0.18	0.10	0.26
Not classifiable (NC)	0.43	0.22	0.28	0.37
All histologies	3.43	2.25	1.85	2.12

* Age-adjusted (1970 United States population) average annual incidence rate per 100,000.

Table 2. Average Annual Incidence Rate of Hodgkin's Disease by Histological Subtype and Social Class for Whites in Los Angeles *

Social Class	NS	MC	LP	LD	NC
High					
1	1.50	1.12	0.47	0.27	0.60
2	1.19	0.66	0.42	0.26	0.27
3	1.23	0.95	0.44	0.25	0.26
4	0.73	0.92	0.18	0.34	0.34
5	0.65	0.55	0.35	0.13	0.35
Low					

* Age-adjusted (1970 United States population) average annual incidence rate per 100,000.

The descriptive epidemiology for NS HD suggests, then, that the causative factors are usually encountered somewhat early in life, with equal frequency among men and women, and more commonly among the well-to-do. Gutensohn and Cole have suggested that this descriptive pattern is consistent with the "paralytic polio" etiologic model.(2) In this model, if a child escapes infection by the causative agent in childhood and does not develop subsequent immunity, he develops a different and more severe disease if infected by the causative agent in adolescence or young adulthood. Risk factors for HD in young adulthood in the United States - small family size, few neighborhood playmates, living in a single family home as a child - are also consistent with this model. While paralytic polio offers a compelling model to "explain" the descriptive epidemiology of young adult HD, other largely unexplored environmental exposures (e.g. exposure to radiation or drugs in utero, childhood, or adolescence) are also consistent with these demographic characteristics.

Along this line, we have conducted two interview case-control studies of HD in the past 10 years (1,3). The only statistically significant risk factor common to both studies was a prior history of amphetamine use. Although the association was apparent at all ages, it was most striking for cases under age 35 at the time of diagnosis (RR=4.0). The mechanism by which amphetamines might relate to the etiology of Hodgkin's disease is not readily apparent. The epidemiology of immunoblastic lymphadenopathy (IBL) may provide a clue. IBL is a distinct pathological lesion which clinically and histologically resembles Hodgkin's disease. The disease may be progressive and some cases become frankly neoplastic. There is evidence that many cases of IBL may be manifest by an idiosyncratic hyperimmune response to drug exposure (4). If drugs or perhaps other foreign antigens can lead to one type of lymphoproliferative disease, it seems possible that a similar mechanism may be involved in Hodgkin's disease.

Not only do the demographic patterns of the non-NS subtypes of HD differ greatly from NS HD, but in general they are similar to those of non-Hodgkin's lymphomas (NHL). For example, as with NHL, the age specific incidence rates for these subtypes tend to increase throughout life and there is no strong association with socioeconomic status. Also, Mexican-Americans have rates of non-NS HD similar to those of other whites. Finally, in Los Angeles there is a clear male excess for the non-NS subtypes, suggesting the possibility that occupational factors play a contributory role.

NON-HODGKIN'S LYMPHOMAS

DESCRIPTIVE EPIDEMIOLOGY

In contrast to the situation for HD, epidemiologic studies of the NHL, including those which have explored demographic factors, have been few. International demographic studies show that there is not as large an international variation for NHL as for many epithelial tumors (5). Low rates, 2-4 times less than those for whites in the US, occur among Japanese living in Japan, but rates for Japanese-Americans more closely resemble those of US whites. In all populations with reliable tumor registries, NHL are primarily diseases of the elderly, although no age is exempt. Rates in males exceed those in females by 30%-100%. Over the past 25 years, there has been an upward trend in NHL incidence, especially in Western countries. Since 1950 in the US, the rate of increase for mortality from NHL has been exceeded only by lung cancer in women and by lung and pancreas cancer in men (6).

A serious handicap in attempting to study the descriptive epidemiology of the NHL is that the broad category of NHL most likely encompasses a heterogeneous group of diseases, each with its own epidemiologic characteristics. Most large tumor registries in the United States, including the Cancer Surveillance Program (CSP), use the International Classification of Diseases for Oncology (ICD-O) (7) to code and tabulate tumor diagnoses, including lymphomas. Based on an international multi-institutional study of over 1000 cases of NHL, a Working Formulation(8) has been proposed as a means of translating the various newly proposed classification systems, such as Lukes-Collins (9), Kiel (10), etc, and of facilitating comparisons of large sets of lymphoma data. In the hope of enhancing the effective use of this system, a group of pathologists and outside consultants from the National Cancer Institute agreed on appropriate assignments of ICD-O code numbers to the Working Formulation (11). This study group then confirmed the prognostic significance of the three major groups in the Working Formulation - low grade, intermediate grade, and high grade lymphomas - on a large data set originally coded to the ICD-O.

Given the prognostic significance of these three major groups of NHL, it seemed possible that these groupings might also have epidemiologic significance. Therefore, we took advantage of this application of ICD-O to the Working Formulation in studying the descriptive epidemiology of the NHL.

In Table 3 are shown the race and sex distributions of these three groups of NHL. Males show an excess over females for each of the three groups. The incidence rates for non Spanish-surnamed whites exceed those of the other racial groups only for the intermediate grade lymphomas. For the high and low grade lymphomas, the highest incidence rates are seen in Spanish-surnamed whites. All three groups are strongly age-related, with incidence rates increasing throughout life, beginning in childhood.

Table 3. Age-adjusted Incidence Rates (Per 100,000) by Race and Sex for High, Intermediate and Low Grade Lymphomas Los Angeles County, 1972-1982.

	High Grade +			Intermediate Grade ++			Low Grade +++		
	Cases	M	F	Cases	M	F	Cases	M	F
Spanish-surnamed	66	0.9	0.7	161	2.3	2.0	406	6.7	4.9
Black	40	0.8	0.3	126	2.4	1.5	248	4.8	3.1
White	332	0.7	0.4	1996	3.5	3.1	3080	6.0	4.5
Japanese	4	0.5	0.3	17	2.0	1.7	46	5.8	3.9
All	452	0.7	0.5	328	3.2	2.9	3855	5.9	4.4

\+ ICD-O 9600, 9602, 9612, 9641, 9750
++ ICD-O 9613-14, 9621-9640, 9642, 9649, 9697-9698
+++ ICD-O 9611, 9620, 9691-9696

The CSP assigns social class on a geographic rather than an individual basis, according to mean income and educational level of the census tract of the case's residence at diagnosis. Incidence of low grade and, especially, intermediate grade lymphomas is related to higher social class in men but not in women; for the high grade lymphomas the opposite is true - the social class association is restricted to women (Table 4).

Table 4. Age-adjusted Incidence Rates (per 100,000) by Social Class and Sex for High, Intermediate, and Low Grade Lymphomas Whites only, Los Angeles County, 1972-1982.

	High Grade		Intermediate Grade		Low Grade	
Social Class	M	F	M	F	M	F
I (High)	0.6	0.9	7.8	5.0	4.7	3.3
II	0.8	0.5	6.5	4.9	3.9	3.7
III	0.5	0.5	5.9	4.4	3.5	3.1
IV	0.6	0.3	4.9	3.8	2.6	2.5
V	1.1	0.3	4.7	5.1	2.8	2.7

Incidence rates for the high grade lymphomas have increased rather dramatically in Los Angeles since 1972. Rates have approximately tripled in men and have more than quadrupled in women. Some of this increase might be artifactual due to changes over time in terminology favored by pathologists. However, there has been no compensatory decline in rates for intermediate and low grade lymphomas; rates for these have remained relatively stable, although there has been a small increase in the incidence rate of low grade lymphomas in women.

This more up to date grouping of the NHL points out a few differences in the demographics of high grade lymphomas. In general, however, it also illustrates the limitations of the major groupings of the Working Formulation in terms of studying etiology.

We have observed a recent change in one other demographic characteristic of NHL which is of special interest. A number of serious infections, immunologic abnormalities and cancers have recently been reported in homosexual males. Originally this syndrome, acquired immune deficiency syndrome (AIDS) was defined to include repeated infections with unusual opportunistic organisms and/or Kaposi's sarcoma (12), but by 1982 it was apparent that the syndrome included other clinical presentations and manitestations, including malignant lymphomas of B lymphocytes (13). These lymphomas have usually been described histologically as immunoblastic sarcomas or small non-cleaved follicular center cell lymphomas both Burkitt and non-Burkitt. Using incidence data from the CSP, we have been able to monitor this purported epidemic of both Kaposi's sarcoma (KS) and malignant lymphoma, and determine its magnitude.

Table 5 looks at incidence data after 1980 in married and never married white men aged 18-54 years for various cancers including Kaposi's sarcoma, non-Hodgkin's lymphoma and several other cancers possibly associated with AIDS (oral cancer, anal cancer, and Hodgkin's disease.) The proportional incidence ratios (PIRS) are equal to the observed number of cases over the expected number times 100, where the expected is based on the average annual number of cases from 1972-1979 for all sites (except lung, which has been decreasing in incidence). The pre-1980 PIR for each site is equal to 100. The category of "never married men" is not synonymous with homosexual men, but it is the closest surrogate available in the registry data. There is little evidence that Hodgkin's disease or anal cancer has increased in either group. Oral cancer in the post 1980 period is 34% greater than expected in never married men although the increase is less in the most recent years. Although AIDS was first identified in 1980, it was not until 1982 that an increase in KS or NHL in young unmarried men first became clearly evident in Los Angeles. The number of cases of KS in this group in 1982 was some 26 times that expected based on pre-1980 rates. There is also a small increase in married men in 1982, based on just 2 cases. The magnitude of the increase in NHL is much less than for KS but still substantial.

Table 5. Proportional Incidence Ratios + Post-1980 for Selected Cancers By Marital Status, Los Angeles County White Males, Ages 18-54

	1980-1982				1982 Only			
Site	Single	(N++)	Married	(N)	Single	(N)	Married	(N)
Kaposi's Sarcoma	1124	(22)	153	(3)	2750	(18)	306	(2)
Non-Hodgkin's Lymphoma	119	(49)	87	(126)	176	(25)	68	(33)
Hodgkin's Disease	104	(73)	90	(73)	112	(27)	82	(22)
Oral Cancer	134	(30)	81	(89)	115	(9)	77	(25)
Anal Cancer	53	(11)	95	(117)	73	(5)	87	(32)

+ Proportional Incidence Ratio = Observed/Expected *100 where expected is based on the average annual incidence for all sites (excluding lung), 1972-1979.
++ N=Number of cases

Table 6 looks at this phenomenon by histology. Since 1980, Burkitt's or Burkitt-like lymphomas have comprised 9% of all non-Hodgkin's lymphomas in young unmarried men in Los Angeles, compared to 1% before 1980. No such proportional increase is apparent in young married men. Similarly, immunoblastic sarcoma has comprised 9% of all NHL in never married men under age 55 since 1980, compared to just 3% before that time.

Table 6. Distribution of Non-Hodgkin's Lymphomas by Histology, Pre- and Post- 1980 Los Angeles County White Males, Ages 18-54

	NEVER MARRIED			MARRIED		
	ALL	BURKITT (B)+B-LIKE	IBS	ALL	B + B-LIKE	IBS
1972-1979	120	1 (1%)	4 (3%)	486	7 (1%)	12 (2%)
1980-1983	91	8 (9%)	8 (9%)	210	3 (1%)	8 (4%)

Analytic Epidemiology

We recently completed a large interview case-control study designed to test multiple hypotheses regarding the etiology of the NHL. The study is population-based and covers approximately a three year period. Controls are neighborhood controls selected by a systematic survey in the neighborhood in which the case lived at diagnosis. Controls are individually matched to cases on date of birth, sex and race. We have attempted to obtain tissue blocks on each interviewed case. Cases are then reviewed and assigned to the Lukes-Collins classification system. Our intent was to determine whether this new functional classification system, which has known clinical and prognostic utility, might also be useful in studying etiology.

It became clear to us early on that it would be useful to look for risk factors not only by individual histologies but also by presenting sites. We originally divided our study into two large parts based on ICD-O coding, one part identifying risk factors for the large cell lymphomas (the so called "histiocytic" lymphomas or "reticulum cell sarcomas" in older classification systems) and the other identifying risk factors for the remaining NHL.

Table 7 shows data for a subcategory of the former group; cases of large cell lymphomas in men diagnosed over a three year period beginning in 1977 and presenting as extranodal primaries of the gastrointestinal tract (stomach, large and small intestine) and oral cavity (tonsil, tongue and pharynx) (14). Cases with clinical or histologic evidence of systemic disease involving these sites were excluded. To put this group in some perspective in terms of size, slightly more than one half of all NHL occur in men, about one-quarter of these are "large cell" and about 20% of these are primary to the gastrointestinal tract or oral cavity. There were 56 such cases during the three year study period, 18 of whom had died before we could reach them. Another 6 refused or their physician refused on their behalf, and 4 others had moved or could not be located. The remaining 28, together with their matched controls, were interviewed using a structured questionnaire which included current and usual, i.e. longest held occupation, and a history of occupational and household chemical exposure obtained by reading a list of potentially hazardous substances and then asking each subject to quantify their exposures. Based on an initial analysis of this subset of cases, asbestos exposure appeared to be strongly associated with risk.

Table 7. Risk Factors for Large Cell Lymphomas of the Gastrointestinal Tract and Oral Cavity

	Discordant pairs (no. cases/no. controls)					
Risk factor	Oral cavity (n=8)	Stomach (n=11)	Intestine (n=9)	Total (n=28)	RR	1-sided p
Asbestos related:						
Usual occupation	2/0	2/1	2/1	6/2	3	0.14
Shipyard work	0/0	4/0	1/0	5/0		0.03
Usual occupation or shipyard work	2/0	4/0	2/1	8/1	8	0.02
Others reporting asbestos exposure	2/1	1/0	2/0	5/1	5	0.11
Any asbestos*	3/0	5/0	4/1	12/1	12	0.002
Malaria	3/0	4/0	3/1	10/1	10	0.006

*By job history or personal report.

For this subgroup of cases, we also conducted a special histologic review. First two hematopathogists reviewed tissue from 26 of the 28 cases independent of any knowledge of chemical exposures and confirmed each to be a lymphoma. A third pathologist with special training in the diagnosis of mesothelioma then reviewed all the gastrointestinal tract cases, including as controls 10 cases originally diagnosed as peritoneal mesotheliomas or undifferentiated carcinomas of the gastrointestinal tract.

We then asked an occupational health physician in our program to review the usual occupations without knowledge as to case or control status, and to categorize persons according to the likelihood of asbestos exposure. For those individuals reporting asbestos exposure, but whose usual occupation did not involve a high potential for asbestos exposure, the circumstances of the exposure were reviewed to determine plausibility of exposure.

Six cases and two controls were judged to have a high likelihood of asbestos exposure based on usual occupation (occupations of cases included two boiler room operators, two shipyard welders, an auto mechanic, and a construction worker whose usual job was to fireproof buildings with asbestos; occupations of controls included a shipwright and an auto mechanic.) Seven other cases and three other controls gave a history of shipyard work at some time in their life. Nine pairs were discordant on asbestos exposure by virtue of shipyard work or usual occupation; eight of these were cases and one was a control. Personal accounts of asbestos exposure constituted a third but less objective measure of asbestos exposure. Five additional cases and one other control gave an occupational history consistent with such exposure. In all, thirteen pairs were discordant on asbestos exposure, and in 12 of these the exposed individual was a case. The median interval between first exposure and disease for the 17 exposed cases was 34 years (range 22-47 years). The median duration of exposure was 19 years; 13 had more than 5 years of exposure, 10 had more than 10 years.

Ten cases and one control gave a history of malaria, which preceded the lymphoma from 24 to 55 years. However only 2 cases and 1 control had malaria in the absence of asbestos exposure, while there were 8 pairs discordant on asbestos without malaria, all of them cases. This suggests the possiblity that the association with malaria may be incidental.

One possible mechanism to explain the relative specificity of this association to the GI tract and oral cavity is that asbestos fibers are ingested and then absorbed by mucosa at these sites. This is true in animals (15) and, since asbestos fibers are found in human urine (16), it is likely true in man. This may precipitate chronic mechanical irritation, resulting in localized stimulation of lymphoid tissue and culminating in the development of a lymphoma. This could be aided by a more systemic effect of asbestos on the immune system since persons with asbestosis display abnormalities of both the humoral and cellular components of the immune system (17, 18).

We had 51 additional pairs of gastrointestinal tract lymphomas in which the case did not have substantial occupational exposure to asbestos (Table 8). Use of certain drugs (antacids, laxatives, and weight loss drugs) was strongly associated with risk. A history of ulcers conveyed high risk, especially for lymphomas of the stomach. There were 10 cases of stomach lymphomas with an ulcer history which preceded the lymphoma diagnosis by at least 2 years, compared to an expected of 4 based on the overall rate of ulcers in controls. Three other cases in this group had a history of either ulcerative colitis or Crohn's disease, with all three primary to the large or small bowel.

Other than the gastrointestinal tract, we have not interviewed enough lymphoma cases for any specific extranodal site to conduct a systematic controlled analysis. Nonetheless, even a casual reading of the questionnaires of these cases, suggests common threads which may account for the site-specificity of their presentation. For example, the case histories of the seven lymphoma cases presenting in the central nervous system, suggests the possibility that heavy systemic corticosteroid therapy (or the indications for such therapy) may have contributed to tumor development (Table 9). A non steroid - related lymphoma of the brain was diagnosed in a young gay male in 1981. The 10 thyroid lymphoma cases also present an interesting pattern. Three cases had a long history of thyroiditis, one of whom could specifically identify his disease as Hashimoto's thyroiditis.

Before looking at some non site-specific preliminary data from the large case-control study, it is worthwhile to review briefly the limited data available from previous epidemiologic research on the NHL.

The relationship between abnormal immune states and high risk of lymphoma has been well documented. Patients with various types of primary immunodeficiency states have an incidence of malignancy some 10,000 times that of the general population. Nearly 60% of these neoplasms are lymphoid in origin (19).

Organ transplant recipients have a 50-100 fold increased risk of NHL. This high risk begins within one year of surgery and the lymphomas which develop in these patients have a striking prediliction for the central nervous system (20). Kinlen has studied the risk of NHL in patients who have been immunosuppressed for other non-malignant conditions (20). While having a much higher than expected risk, the observed risk is substantially less than in organ transplant patients, suggesting that immunostimulation by the graft enhances the high risk state created by immunosuppression alone.

Finally, an association between the autoimmune/connective tissue complex of diseases, for example, rheumatoid arthritis, systemic lupus erythematosis and Sjogren's syndrome, has been described (21-23). However, only a very small fraction of lymphoma cases report such disorders and, in the various case series, the lymphomas often precede the development of the autoimmune disorder. The most likely hypothesis for their coexistence is an underlying deficiency of the immune system conveying susceptibility to both disease processes.

Table 8. Risk Factors for Non-Asbestos Associated Gastrointestinal Trac Lymphomas +

Risk Factor	Discordant Pairs	RR	P
Drugs ++			
Weight Loss Drugs	15	14.0	<0.01
Antacids	23	2.3	0.06
Laxatives	7	6.0	0.06
Medical History			
Ulcer	20	1.9	0.18
Ulcerative Colitis/Crohn's	3		0.08
Chemical Exposures			
Metal Dusts	8	3.0	0.16

\+ Stomach, small and large intestines (n=51)
++ Continuous daily use for at least two months.

Table 9. Extranodal Lymphomas of the Brain: Exposures/Characteristics of Possible Etiologic Significance

Age	Sex	Race	Exposures/Characteristics
62	F	W	Cancer Age 43-Radiation, Prednisone
53	M	W	Systemic Steroids Age 48 Colon Cancer Age 50 Machinist-Oil Refinery (Solvents)
40	M	W	Gay
72	F	W	Severe Skin Allergies: ?Systemic Steroids Riveter-Aircraft Industry (Metal Dusts)
47	M	W	Asthma
57	F	W	Severe Skin Allergies: Systemic Steroids
46	F	W	Dilantin Age 43 Vitamin A-Megadoses

One histopathologic type of non-Hodgkin's lymphoma that has been relatively well studied epidemiologically is Burkitt's lymphoma (BL). sporadic cases of BL occur throughout the world but the disease is endemic in Papua, New Guinea and in tropical Africa. Several features of BL make it unique among the NHL. In endemic areas, BL commonly occurs in childhood and commonly involves the jaw as the primary site. Based in part on sero-epidemiologic data, BL appears to be closely linked with infection by Epstein-Barr virus, and the pattern of occurrence shows remarkably close geographic correlation with that of endemic malaria (24).

One of the difficulties in analyzing our large case-control study of NHL is determining an appropriate method for grouping cases according to histology. In our pathologic review of slides from the interviewed cases, we have assigned cases to the Lukes-Collins classification system. Since ICD-O rubrics include terminology from all the new functional classification systems, a new ICD-O code was assigned to each case based on the Lukes-Collins terminology. Our first approach to grouping cases by histology was again to utilize the cross-classification of ICD-O rubrics to the Working Formulation, and assign cases into high, intermediate and low grade categories, realizing that there are distinct morphologic and functional "types" of lymphomas within each grade that will need to be explored in detail. The final two tables give examples of the types of data we are able to generate from this study, overall and for individual histologies.

Certain diseases that, a priori, we thought might relate to risk overall, such as rheumatoid arthritis and mononucleosis, were not significantly associated with risk of NHL (Table 10). History of tonsillectomy or appendectomy did not convey high risk. A history of ulcerative colitis was strongly associated with risk, although the number of cases with this history was small. Only two persons in the study had a history of systemic lupus erythematosis, both cases. A personal cancer history increased risk by 70%. We are in the process of looking at the site distribution of these cancers. Having a first degree relative with hodgkin's disease or a non-Hodgkin's lymphoma more than doubled risk. However, we do not have an independent medical confirmation of these familial cases.

Table 10. Risk Factors for Non-Hodgkin's Lymphomas: A Preliminary Analysis of 700 Pairs

Risk Factor-Health History	Discordant Pairs	RR	P
Self:			
Mononucleosis	31	1.4	NS
Ulcerative Colitis	19	2.8	0.04
Asthma	87	0.9	NS
Rheumatoid Arthritis	36	0.9	NS
Diabetis	66	0.9	NS
Cancer	147	1.7	<0.01
"Shingles"	92	1.0	NS
Tonsillectomy	278	1.2	NS
Appendectomy	240	1.2	NS
Smoking	270	0.9	NS
First Degree Relative:			
Hodgkin's Disease/Lymphoma	50	2.3	<0.01
Rheumatoid Arthritis	128	1.4	NS

The final table looks at risk factors for 100 pairs of "high grade" lymphomas, nearly two thirds of which are immunoblastic sarcomas (Table 11). A history of herpes zoster and malaria were significantly associated with this group of lymphomas, associations not apparent for the entire series of 700 pairs. The diagnosis of herpes zoster in the cases preceded the lymphoma diagnosis by a minimum of 2 years and a median of 8 years. Non-incidental regular occupational benzene and asbestos exposure were more strongly associated with the high grade lymphomas than for all NHL, although only the latter association was statistically significant.

Table 11. Risk Factors for "High Grade" Lymphomas: A Preliminary Analysis of 100 Pairs +

Risk Factor	Discordant Pairs	RR	P
Medical History			
Malaria	7	6.0	0.06
"Shingles"	16	3.0	0.05
Rheumatoid Arthritis	5	0.7	NS
Ulcerative Colitis	4	3.0	NS
Diabetis	9	1.3	NS
Tonsillectomy	38	1.4	NS
Appendectomy	30	1.5	NS
Smoking	32	0.9	NS
Occupational Exposures			
Benzene	9	3.5	0.10
Metal Dusts	26	1.6	NS
Asbestos	24	2.4	0.04

+ 65 cases are histologically "Immunoblastic Sarcomas"

REFERENCES:

1. Henderson BE, Dworsky R, Pike MC, et al: Risk factors for nodular sclerosis and other types of Hodgkin's disease. Cancer Res 39:4507, 1979.
2. Gutensohn N, Cole P: Epidemiology of Hodgkin's disease in the young. Int J Cancer 19:545, 1977.
3. Newell G, Rawlings W, Kinnear BR, et al: Case control study of Hodgkin's disease. I. Results of the interview questionnaire. JNCI 51:1437, 1973.
4. Lukes RJ, Tindle BH: Immunoblastic lymphadenopathy - a hyperimmune entity resembling Hodgkin's disease. N Eng J Med 292:1, 1975.
5. Correa P, O'Conor GT: Geographic pathology of lymphoreticular tumors: Summary of survey from the geographic pathology committee of the International Union Against Cancer. JNCI 50:1609, 1973.
6. Cantor KP, Fraumeni JF: Geographic and temporal patterns of non-Hodgkin's lymphoma mortality in US counties, 1950-1975. Cancer Res 40:2645, 1980.
7. World Health Organization: International Classification of Diseases for Oncology. WHO, Geneva, Switzerland, 1976.
8. National Cancer Institute: Study of classifications of non-Hodgkin's lymphomas; summary and description of a working formulation for clinical usage. Cancer 49:2112, 1982.
9. Lukes RJ, Collins RD: New approaches to the classification of lymphomas. Brit J Cancer 31, Supplement 11:1, 1975.
10. Gerald-Merchant R, Hamlin I, Lennert K, et al: Classification of non-Hodgkin's lymphomas. Lancet 2:406, 1974.

11. Percy C, O'Conor G, Ries LG, Jaffe E: Non-Hodgkin's lymphomas: Application of the international classification of diseases for oncology (ICD-O) to the working formulation: Cancer 54:1435, 1984.
12. Friedman-Klein A, Laubenstein L, Marmor M, et al: Kaposi's sarcoma and pneumocystis pneumonia among homosexual men - New York City and California. MMWR 30:305, 1981.
13. Ziegler JL, Drew WL, Miner RC, et al: Outbreak of Burkitt's-like lymphoma in homosexual men. Lancet ii:631, 1982.
14. Ross RK, Dworsky R, Nichols P, et al: Gastrointestinal tract lymphomas and occupational exposure to asbestos. Lancet ii:1118, 1982.
15. Sebastien P, Masse R, Bignon J: Recovery of ingested asbestos fibers from the gastrointestinal lymph in rats. Environ Res 22:201, 1980.
16. Cook PM, Olson GF: Ingested mineral fibers: elimination in human urine. Science 204:195, 1979.
17. Kagan E, Soloman A, Cochrane JC, et al: Immunological studies of patients with asbestosis. I. Studies of cell-mediated immunity. Clin Exp Immunol 28:261, 1977.
18. Kagan E, Solomon A, Cochrane JC, et al: Immunological studies of patients with asbestosis. I. Studies of circulatory lymphoid cell numbers and of humoral immunity. Clin Exp Immunol 28:268, 1977.
19. Gatti RA, Good RA: Occurrence of malignancy in immunodeficiency diseases: A literature review. Cancer 28:89, 1971.
20. Kinlen LJ, Shiel ALR, Peto J, et al: A collaborative study of cancer in patients who have received immunosuppressive therapy. Brit Med J 2:1461, 1979.
21. Isomaki HA, Hakulnen T, Joutsenlahti U: Excess risk of lymphomas, leukemia and myeloma in patients with rheumatoid arthritis. J Chronic Dis 31:691, 1978.
22. Wyburn-Mason R: SLE and lymphoma, Lancet i:156, 1979.
23. Kassan SS, Thomas JL, Moutsopoulos HM: Increased risk of lymphoma in sicca syndrome. Ann Intern Med 89:888, 1978.
24. Morrow RH: Burkitt's lymphoma. In: Schottenfeld D, Fraumeni JF (eds) Cancer Epidemiology and Prevention. W B Saunders Co., Philadelphia: p. 779, 1982.

CLINICO-EPIDEMIOLOGICAL FEATURES OF ADULT T-CELL LEUKEMIA/LYMPHOMA (ATLL) IN JAPAN: RELATIONS OF HTLV-I/ATLV INFECTION TO ATLL MANIFESTATION

KAZUO TAJIMA AND SUKETAMI TOMINAGA

INTRODUCTION

The age-adjusted death rate of malignant lymphomas in the Kyushu district including Okinawa Prefecture, the southern-most district in Japan, was twice as high as those for other districts of Japan.[1] A nationwide survey[2] showed that the excess rate of mortality from malignant lymphomas in Kyushu was due to the high incidence of adult T-cell leukemia/lymphoma (ATLL).[3] The Kyushu district seemed to be the most typical endemic area of ATLL in the world. It was estimated that more than 300 new cases of ATLL will occur every year in the Kyushu district. In addition to the Kyushu district, many cases of ATLL have been observed in other districts of Japan[2] and in the northern part of Taiwan.[4] It was reported[5] that cases similar to Japanese ATLL were found among Caribbean people who might have originated in central Africa.

In 1980 human T-cell leukemia virus (HTLV/HTLV-I), which is etiologically associated with ATLL, was isolated from the cultivated tumor cells of patients with ATLL.[6,7] Independently of HTLV, the same virus, called adult T-cell leukemia virus (ATLV) was identified in the ATLL cell lines MT1 and MT2 in 1981.[8,9] The sera of most, if not all, cases of ATLL were shown to be HTLV-associated antigen-reactive.[8,10] Furthermore, positive reactivity to HTLV in sera was commonly observed among healthy adults in the ATLL-endemic areas in Japan[11-13] (see Table 1).

In the present paper, we review clinico-pathological and epidemiological findings of ATLL in Japan and discuss the epidemiological aspects of the relationship between HTLV infection and the ATLL manifestation in the Kyushu district.

Table 1. Positive rate of anti-HTLV antibody in sera among patients with ATLL and blood donors from 40 to 64 years of age in Kyushu and other districts.

Subjects	Kyushu district Positive/Tested (%)		Other districts Positive/Tested (%)	
ATLL patients	115/115	(100.0)	34/40	(85.0)
Blood donors	241/3026	(8.0)	95/12,090	(0.8)

Data source: T- and B-Cell Malignancy Study Group, 1984;[10] Maeda et al, 1984.[13]

CLINICO-PATHOLOGICAL FEATURES OF ATLL IN JAPAN

The analysis of the clinical data on admission in the 300 ATLL cases collected by the T- and B-Cell Malignancy Study Group throughout Japan from 1980-1984[2,10] showed marked characteristics in the clinico-pathological features as follows: (1) the onset in adulthood with the mean age of 53 years and the main age distribution group of 50-59 years; (2) a relatively small male/female ratio of 1.3; (3) frequent leukemic manifestation (80%), generalized lymphadenopathy (70%), hepatosplenomegaly (30%) and skin involvement (30%); (4) frequent hypercalcemia (30%, >5.5mEq/l), eosinophilia (10%, >5%), thrombocytopenia (20%, <100,000/mm^3), hypogammaglobulinemia (40%, <1000mg/dl), elevated lactate dehydrogenase (40%, >1000IU); (5) negative purified protein derivatives skin test (75%); (6) neoplastic cells with helper T-cell character (OKT4 positive) and peculiar pleomorphic nuclei (convoluted); (7) rapid clinical course with 50% survival time of less than six months; (8) a family history of lymphoid malignancies and cancer of other sites.

GEOGRAPHICAL DISTRIBUTION OF ATLL AND HTLV-CARRIERS IN JAPAN

It was revealed[2,3,10] that most patients with ATLL were from the Kyushu district (see Figure 1). It is noted that the increased incidence of ATLL found in the metropolitan areas, such as Tokyo and Osaka, is found in the rural coastal areas in the Kyushu district. According to the Vital Statistics Japan Series,[15] the patients with malignant lymphomas were mainly clustered in the Kyushu district, particularly in the rural areas of the four prefectures, Nagasaki, Miyazaki, Kagoshima and Okinawa (see Figure 2). The death rates of malignant lymphomas in some islands in

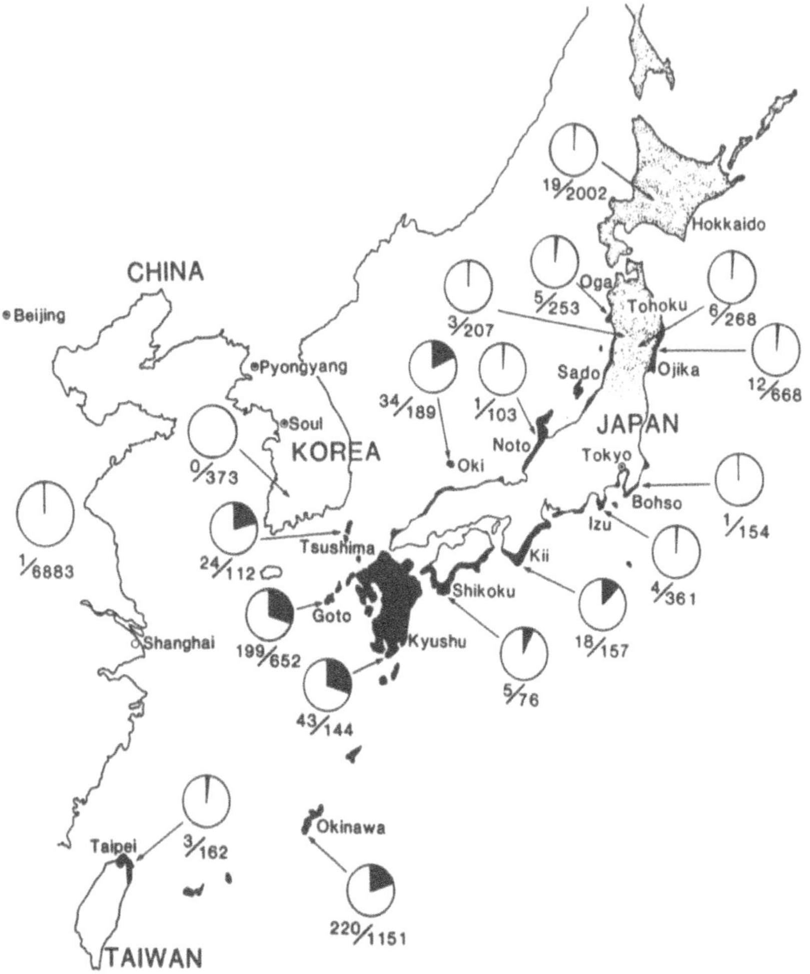

FIGURE 1. Geographical distribution of patients with ATLL and HTLV-carrier adults in Japan, China, Korea and Taiwan. Black areas correspond to the endemic areas of ATLL. In stippled areas of Hokkaido and Tohoku districts, patients with ATLL have been found sporadically. Figures under circles indicate the number of positives/tested subjects of anti-HTLV antibody.

Data source: T- and B-Cell Malignancy Study Group, 1981[2] and 1984;[10] Hinuma et al, 1983;[11] Tajima and Hinuma, 1984;[14] and Zeng et al, 1984.[19]

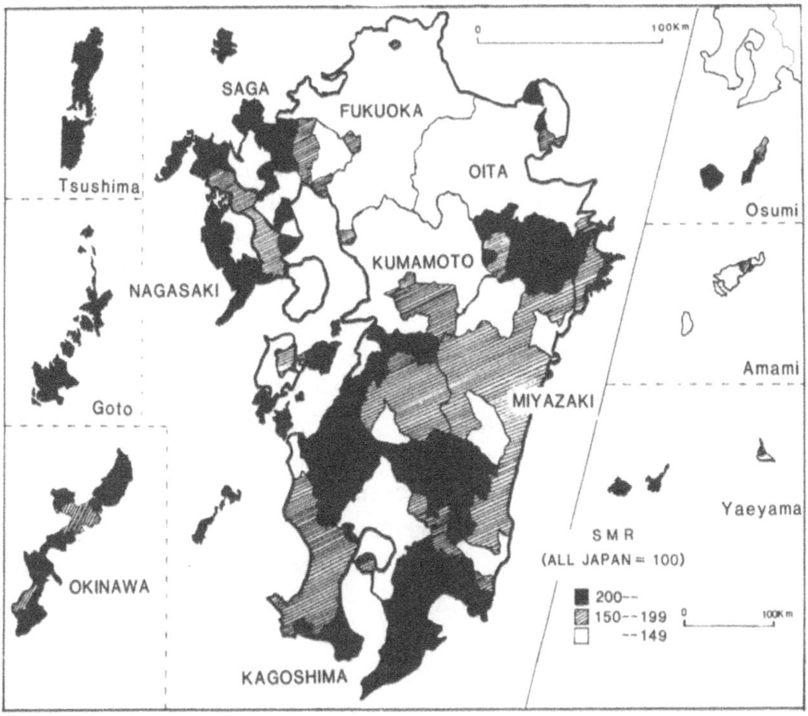

FIGURE 2. Geographical comparison of standardized mortality ratio (SMR) of malignant lymphomas (ICDs, 200-202) by city and county in the Kyushu district in 1978-1982.

these prefectures were four to six times as high as that for all Japan.

Besides the Kyushu district, ATLL patients were observed at the coastal areas in Japan, such as south Shikoku, Kii, Izu, Bohso, Ojika, Oki, Noto, Sado, Oga and others along the Pacific Ocean and Japan Sea (see Figure 1). In Hokkaido and Tohoku districts, however, ATLL cases were sporadically observed even in the mountainous areas.[2,10] It is interesting that the geographical distribution of ATLL patients in the northern part of Japan seemed to be rather different from that in the other districts. In addition, several cases of ATLL were observed among Chinese people[5] in the northern part of Taiwan, where many Japanese had immigrated, probably from the Kyushu district, and had lived for several decades before the end of World War II.

A high incidence of anti-HTLV antibody-positive persons was found in the Kyushu district where the incidence of ATLL was markedly high.[11-13] Subjects with anti-HTLV titers more than 1:5 dilution of sera were regarded as so-called HTLV carriers, based on the observation that HTLV antigen could be regularly found in short-term cultures of lymphocytes from anti-HTLV-positive subjects.[16,17] From a nationwide seroepidemiological survey of HTLV,[11,14] it was shown that the geographical distribution of HTLV carriers closely correlated with that of patients with ATLL (see Figure 1).

Outside Japan in the southeast Asian countries, HTLV carriers were observed among Chinese in the northern part of Taiwan, where a few cases of ATLL have been found.[5,18] In Korea and mainland China, however, no HTLV carriers have been observed among several thousands adults, except for one Chinese woman whose husband was a Japanese HTLV carrier, immigrated from the Kyushu district 40 years previously.[19] It was strongly suspected that this Chinese woman had been infected with HTLV from her Japanese husband.

EPIDEMIOLOGICAL FEATURES OF HTLV

It was reported[12,20] that the prevalence of HTLV carriers among healthy persons in the ATLL-endemic areas increased with age, especially in females (see Table 2). It is interesting that positive rates of anti-HTLV for children were low even in the endemic area.[12] From the epidemiological analysis on the familial distribution of HTLV carriers in the Goto Islands, which are typical ATLL-endemic areas and located 100km west of Nagasaki City in the Kyushu district (see Figures 1 and 2), two main routes of

Table 2. Age- and sex-specific positive rate of anti-HTLV antibody among 840 healthy adults of four villages in the Goto Islands

Age (Years)	Positive rate (%) in males (Positive/Tested)		Positive rate (%) in females (Positive/Tested)	
20-39	11.0	(9/82)	9.4	(8/85)
40-59	22.1	(34/154)	27.8	(65/234)
60-	24.6	(28/114)	41.5	(71/171)
Total	20.3	(71/350)	29.4	(144/490)
40-	23.1	(62/268)	33.6	(136/405)

Data source: Tajima et al, 1984.[20]

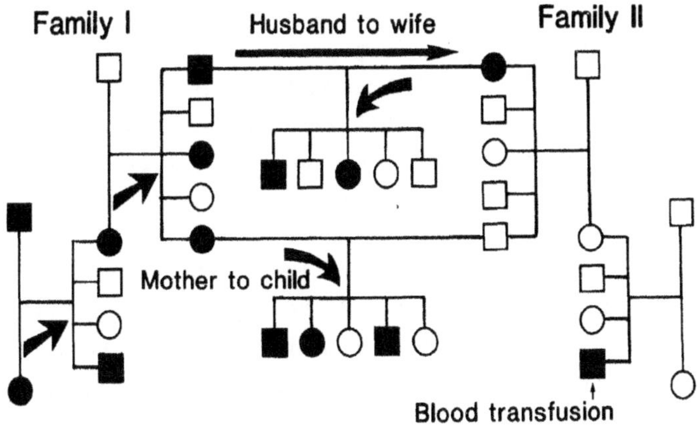

FIGURE 3. Three main routes of HTLV-transmission. Squares and circles indicate males and females respectively, and black indicates HTLV-carriers in supposed pedigrees of family I (HTLV carriers) and family II (non-carriers).

natural transmission of HTLV were suggested[12,14,20] (see Figure 3): (1) vertical or horizontal transmission from carrier-mother to child; more than 40% of children over 20 years were infected with HTLV in this way; (2) horizontal transmission between spouses, especially from carrier-husband to wife. More than 80% (32/38) of wives with carrier-husbands over age 40 were infected with HTLV, but only 19% (28/245) of wives with noncarrier husbands were infected; this figure was almost the same as the carrier rate of total husbands (see Table 3). On the contrary, uninfected wives with carrier-husbands over 40 years were very few. The higher incidence of HTLV infection in females in the higher age group seemed to be related to the one-way transmission (from husband to wife) of HTLV after marriage.

Table 3. Distribution of anti-HTLV positives among husbands and wives according to the anti-HTLV positivity of spouses

Anti-HTLV positivity	Age group of spouses 40-59	60 +	Total
Wife(+)/Husband(+)	21/27 (78)	11/11 (100)	32/38 (84)
Wife(+)/Husband(-)	16/94 (17)	12/51 (24)	28/145 (19)
Husband(+)/Wife(+)	22/32 (69)	13/31 (42)	35/63 (56)
Husband(+)/Wife(-)	5/75 (7)	1/54 (2)	6/129 (5)

Figures in parentheses indicate the positive rate (%) of anti-HTLV antibody in each group.

Recently, lymphocytes with HTLV antigen were identified from breast milk of carrier-mother,[21] which suggests that HTLV could be transmitted from mother to child through breast milk besides through placenta. Futhermore, HTLV antigens were identified from lymphocytes in semen of carrier-husbands,[22] which suggests some possibility that HTLV could be naturally transmitted from husband to wife through semen.

Other than natural transmission, parenteral infection mainly by whole blood transfusion is one of the important transmissible routes of HTLV. More than 60% of noncarrier recipients were infected with HTLV after transfusion of anti-HTLV-positive blood.[23]

GENETICAL BACKGROUND OF HTLV CARRIERS

It was revealed[2,10,11] that HTLV carriers and ATLL patients were clustered in the rural areas which had long been separated from urbanized city or town. Besides geographical clustering, intrafamilial clustering of HTLV carriers was observed which corresponded to the familial aggregation of patients with ATLL.[24] Even though familial aggregation itself may not necessarily signify the effect of genetic factors, it seems worthwhile to search for the common backgrounds of HTLV carriers and ATLL patients. As a preliminary study on this matter, the distribution of HLA-A, -B and -C antigens between HTLV carriers and noncarriers among inhabitants in the two villages of the ATLL-endemic areas were compared. However, no consistent relationship between HLA types and HTLV carriers was observed, which did not support the possibility of the existence of individuals who were genetically susceptible to HTLV infection.[25]

CHRONOLOGICAL CHANGES OF HTLV INFESTATION IN KYUSHU

It was revealed[11,12,14,20] that the frequency of anti-HTLV antibody-positive individuals in the ATLL-endemic areas increases with age, especially in females, but is very low among the younger generation of both sexes, even in the ATLL-endemic areas. It was strongly suggested that HTLV is naturally transmitted from mother to child vertically or horizontally. However, antibody to HTLV in children who have been naturally infected with HTLV at an early age may not be expressed because of a small amount of antigen and/or suppression of antibody production by immuno-tolerance in childhood. Sero-conversion may occur in later life with repeated stimulation by augmented HTLV antigen in the host. In the recent studies, however, it was suggested that sero-positivity against HTLV antigen among individuals in the ATLL-endemic areas was consistent by time for several years and sero-conversion was seen in very few exceptional cases (unpublished data). Meanwhile, HTLV antigen was not isolated by in vitro culture of leukocytes from antibody-negative children whose mothers were HTLV carriers.[26] Furthermore, it has been reported that the positive rate for anti-HTLV among school children has been decreasing during the past several years according to the results of retrospective sero-epidemiological studies in the Goto Islands.[27]

Sero-epidemiological studies on filariasis and HTLV infection[28,29] suggested that the incidence of filarial infection positively correlated with HTLV infection among inhabitants in the Goto Islands, where filariasis had been endemic up until 20 years ago (see Table 4). In recent years, however, filariasis has become rare due to the introduction of preventive measures. In addition, the poor nutritional condition in these ATLL-endemic areas in the past has been remarkably improved over the last 20 to 30 years, which may serve as a prevention against natural HTLV infection in the host.

From these epidemiological evidences, it is presumable that the incidence of HTLV carriers by natural transmission is declining at present, which may be one reason why positive rates of anti-HTLV were very low in the young generation and increased with age.

Table 4. Comparison of the positive rate of anti-HTLV antibody between low and high filaria-antibody titer groups in persons over age 40 in the Goto Islands

Anti-filaria antibody titer	Anti-HTLV antibody: Males Positives/Subjects (%)	Anti-HTLV antibody: Females Positives/Subjects (%)
Low ($\leq 2^{0.5}$)	8/72 (11.1)	30/115 (26.1)
High ($\geq 2^{1.0}$)	16/44 (36.4)	42/78 (53.8)
Total	24/116 (20.7)	72/193 (37.3)

Data source: Tajima et al, 1983.[29]

INCIDENCE OF ATLL PATIENTS AMONG HTLV CARRIERS IN KYUSHU

Table 5 shows estimated death rates of T-cell lymphoma and non-T-cell lymphoma in adults over age 20 in Kyushu and other districts, which were calculated respectively from the death rates of non-Hodgkin lymphoma in 1979-1981[15] and the proportional incidence of T-cell and non-T-cell lymphoma in both districts in recent years.[10] The death rate of non-T-cell lymphoma in the Kyushu district was basically the same as that of other districts, but the rate of T-cell lymphoma was markedly high in the Kyushu district, due to the high incidence of ATLL. It was supposed that the death rate of the ordinal type of lymphomas in the Kyushu district was not so different from that in the other districts. Therefore, an estimated death rate of ATLL among adults in the Kyushu district in 1979-1981 was 4.3/100,000, computed from the difference in the death rates between Kyushu and other districts. Since the vast majority of patients with ATLL probably died within a year, the death rate of ATLL could correspond to the incidence rate of ATLL in the Kyushu district. Recently, we estimated that the annual death rate from ATLL in the Kyushu district was 350 (200 in males and 150 in females) in 1978-1982, and 500 to 600 thousand HTLV carriers might exist in the Kyushu district in recent years. Furthermore, the annual incidence rate of ATLL among HTLV carriers over age 40 was estimated at 78/100,000, but it was only 15/100,000 in the younger generation, age 20-39 years (unpublished data).

Meanwhile, in the Goto Islands crude death rates for individuals over age 40 with non-Hodgkin lymphoma were 41.7/100,000 in males and 22.3/100,000 in females, four times higher than those

Table 5. Estimated death rate of T-cell and non-T-cell lymphoma in adults older than 20 years in the Kyushu and other districts in 1979-1981.

District	T-cell type lymphoma (%)	non-T-cell type lymphoma (%)	Total (%)
Kyushu	6.01 (78)	1.70 (22)	7.71 (100)
Other districts	1.61 (47)	1.81 (53)	3.42 (100)

Figures in parentheses indicate the proportion of T- and non-T-cell lymphoma in non-Hodgkin's lymphoma.

Data source: T- and B-Cell Malignancy Study Group, 1984.[10]

of all Japan (9.0 and 5.2) in 1978-1982. The recent incidence rate for ATLL in the Goto Islands was estimated at 32.7 in males and 17.1 in females. In order to estimate the annual incidence rate of ATLL among HTLV carriers in the Goto Islands, the estimated number of ATLL cases and HTLV carriers were calculated first. The estimated number of deaths from ATLL in the Goto Islands is shown in Table 6. Vital statistics of cancer deaths in Japan were based on the records of the death certificates written by the physician in charge when a patient died, and some cases of ATLL might be missed in the Goto Islands due to inadequate medical facilities. Therefore, more than 10 cases of ATLL (six in males and four in females) might have occurred in a year in the Goto Islands recently. Next, the estimated number of HTLV carriers over age 40 in the Goto Islands was calculated from the data of age-specific positive rates of anti-HTLV antibody among inhabitants in the Goto Islands (see Table 6). It was suggested that about 12,000 HTLV carriers (4,000 males and 8,000 females) over age 40 might exist in the Goto Islands in recent years. From these data, the annual incidence rate of ATLL among 1,000 HTLV carriers over age 40 was estimated to be 1.4 in males, 0.5 in females, and 0.8 in both sexes, similar figures to those for all of Kyushu district. Previously we estimated the death rates of ATLL among the same subjects in the Goto Islands at 0.9 in males and 0.3 in females. These figures were slightly lower than those in the present paper,

Table 6. Estimated death rate for ATLL among HTLV carriers over age 40 in the Goto Islands in 1978-1982

Age (Years)	Estimated # of deaths from ATLL*			Estimated # of HTLV carriers**			Estimated death rate among 1,000 HTLV carriers		
	Male	Female	Total	Male	Female	Total	Male	Female	Total
40-59	2.51	1.58	4.09	2,700	3,860	6,560	0.93	0.41	0.62
60-	3.74	2.50	6.24	1,700	4,140	5,840	2.20	0.60	1.07
Total	6.25	4.08	10.33	4,400	8,000	12,400	1.42	0.51	0.83

*Differences between the observed number of deaths and the expected number of deaths from non-Hodgkin's lymphoma in the Goto Islands in 1978-1982.

**Calculated from the age-specific positive rate of anti-HTLV antibody in Table 2.

because the number of deaths from ATLL was underestimated in the previous report.[20]

POSSIBLE RISK TIME OF HTLV INFECTION FOR ATLL MANIFESTATION

It seems that HTLV infection is etiologically a main causative agent of ATLL manifestation. All patients with ATLL in the Kyushu district had antibody to HTLV antigen,[4] and the proviral genome was always detected in the chromosomal DNA of the leukemia cells.[9] Recent analysis of the complete nucleotide sequence of HTLV genome indicates that HTLV has no homology with the normal human genome,[30] and the transformation mechanism of T cells by HTLV infection has not yet been clarified. It is interesting, however, that the region between the env gene and 3'LTR, named pX gene, codes for 10,000-27,000 dalton polypeptides, and these peptides may play an important role in transformation of HTLV-infected T cells.[30]

From the sero-epidemiological evidences, the age and geographical distribution of HTLV carriers strongly correlated with that of patients with ATLL,[2,10,11,14] and sero-conversion against HTLV infection precedes the manifestation of ATLL.[31] However, the estimated death rates of ATLL were relatively low, eg, 0.5 in females and 1.4 in males among 1,000 HTLV carriers over age 40, even in the ATLL-endemic areas. These figures are smaller than those of stomach cancer for the same period among the same age group of the general population in Japan.

According to a nationwide survey, most of the patients with ATLL who have been observed in metropolitan areas were raised in the ATLL-endemic areas. These patients had been infected with HTLV in childhood from mothers of HTLV carriers. HTLV is horizontally transmitted from husband to wife, and the incidence of HTLV carriers increased in females over age 50.[12,14] However, ATLL is more common in males than in females over age 50.[2,10] This discrepancy of the trends in the sex ratio between HTLV carriers and ATLL patients might be explained by the fact that the first infection with HTLV in adulthood, such as natural infection from husband to wife, may rarely lead to development of ATLL.

In Japan, blood transfusion has become applicable to medical treatment since 1950, and the system of blood centers has widely progressed and developed throughout Japan. Therefore, many HTLV carriers have been generated for the last several decades by whole blood transfusion, not only in the Kyushu district but in other districts. According to the nationwide case-control study on risk factors for ATLL, no positive relationship between ATLL manifestation and a history of blood transfusion was observed.[10]

It was suggested from this epidemiological evidence that average latent time of ATLL was 40-50 years or longer, since there could be a critical age range in which HTLV infection leads to ATLL manifestation, possibly in childhood or in an early stage when T lymphocytes are still differentiated and mature in the thymic gland under the influence of various antigens.

CONCLUSION

HTLV carriers and patients with ATLL were primarily distributed in limited zones in Japan. Besides geographical clustering, an intrafamilial aggregation of HTLV carriers was observed as seen in ATLL cases. HTLV carriers increased with age, especially in females. HTLV is naturally transmitted from mother to child vertically or horizontally and from husband to wife horizontally. Other than natural transmission, HTLV is tranmitted by whole-blood transfusion from carrier-donor to noncarrier-recipient. It is assumed that incidence of HTLV infection by natural transmission among younger generations is declining in recent years. It was estimated that the number of HTLV carriers was 500,000 to 600,000, and annual incidence of ATLL was 350 in the Kyushu district. Estimated incidence rate of ATLL among 1,000 HTLV carriers over age 40 was 1.4 in males and 0.5 in females. It was suggested that average latent time of ATLL was 40 to 50 years after HTLV infection in a critical age range, possibly in childhood or more early stage. In order to clarify the above epidemiological evidences in more detail and to conduct plans for prevention of ATLL, a vast epidemiological study on risk factors for HTLV infection and ATLL manifestation (supported by grant-in-aid for Cancer Research from the Ministry of Health and Welfare) is now underway.

REFERENCES

1. Tajima K, Tominaga S, Kuroishi T, Shimizu H, Suchi H. 1979. Geographical features and epidemiological approach to endemic T-cell leukemia/lymphoma in Japan. Jpn J Clin Oncol 9:495-504.
2. The T- and B-cell Malignancy Study Group. Statistical analysis

of immunologic, clinical and histopathologic data on lymphoid malignancies in Japan. Jpn J Clin Oncol 11:15-38.
3. Uchiyama T, Yodoi J, Sagawa W, Takatsuki K, Uchino H. 1977. Adult T-cell leukemia: clinical and hematologic features of 16 cases. Blood 50:481-492.
4. Pan I-H (personal communication).
5. Catovsky D, Greaves MF, Rose M, Galton DAG, Goolden AWG, McClusky DR, White JM, Lampert I, Bourikas G, Ireland R, Brownell AI, Bridges JM, Blattner WA, Gallo RC. 1982. Adult T-cell lymphoma-leukaemia in blacks from the West Indies. Lancet 1:639-643.
6. Poiesz BJ, Ruscetti FW, Gazdar AF, Bunn PA, Minna JD, Gallo RC. 1980. Detection and isolation of type C retrovirus particles from fresh and cultured lymphocytes of a patient with cutaneous T-cell lymphoma. Proc Natl Acad Sci USA 77:7415-7419.
7. Reitz MS, Poiesz BJ, Ruscetti FW, Gallo RC. 1981. Characterization and distribution of nucleic acid sequences of a novel type C retrovirus isolated from neoplastic human T lymphocytes. Proc Natl Acad Sci USA 78:1887-1891.
8. Hinuma Y, Nagata K, Hanaoka M, Nakai M, Matsumoto T, Kinoshita K, Shirakawa S, Miyoshi I. 1981. Adult T-cell leukemia: antigen in an ATL cell line and detection of antibodies to the antigen in human sera. Proc Natl Acad Sci USA 78:6476-6480.
9. Yoshida M, Miyoshi I, Hinuma Y. 1982. Isolation and characterization of retrovirus from cell lines of human adult T-cell leukemia and its implication in the disease. Proc Natl Acad Sci USA 79:2031-2035.
10. T- and B-cell Malignancy Study Group. Clinical and epidemiological findings of adult T-cell leukemia/lymphoma in Japan: a nation-wide study II. (unpublished)
11. Hinuma Y, Komoda H, Chosa T, Kondo T, Kohakura M, Takenaka T, Kikuchi M, Ichimaru M, Yunoki K, Sato I, Matsuo R, Takiuchi Y, Uchino H, Hanaoka M. 1982. Antibodies on adult T-cell leukemia-virus-associated antigen (ATLA) in sera from patients with ATL and controls in Japan: a nation-wide sero-epidemiological study. Int J Cancer 29:631-635.
12. Tajima K, Tominaga S, Suchi T, Kawagoe T, Komoda H, Hinuma Y, Oda T, Fujita K. 1982. Epidemiological analysis of the distribution of antibody to adult T-cell leukemia-virus-associated antigen: possible horizontal transmission of adult T-cell leukemia virus. Gann Monogr Cancer Res 73:893-901.
13. Maeda Y, Furukawa M, Takehara Y,, Yoshimura K, Miyamoto K, Matsuura T, Morishima Y, Tajima K, Okochi K, Hinuma Y. 1984. Prevalence of possible adult T-cell leukemia virus-carriers among volunteer blood donors in Japan: a nation-wide study. Int J Cancer 33:717-720.
14. Tajima K, Hinuma Y. 1984 (in press). Epidemiological features of adult T-cell leukemia virus. In: Pathological Aspects of Cancer Epidemiology: Immunological, Virological, Endocrinological and Genetical Factors.
15. Ministry of Health and Welfare. Vital Statistics Japan Series, Vol 2, 1978-1982.
16. Hinuma Y, Gotoh Y, Sugamura K, Nagata K, Gotoh T, Nakai N, Kamada N, Matsumoto T, Kinoshita K. 1982. A retrovirus associated with human adult T-cell leukemia: in vitro activation. Gann 73:341-344.
17. Gotoh Y, Sugamura K, Hinuma Y. 1982. Healthy carriers of a human retrovirus, adult T-cell leukemia virus (ATLV): demonstration by clonal culture of ATLV-carrying T cells from peri-

pheral blood. Proc Natl Acad Sci USA 79:4780-4782.
18. Hinuma Y, Chosa T, Komoda H, Mori I, Suzuki T, Tajima K, Pan I-H, Lee M. 1983. Spradic retrovirus (ATLV)-seropositive individuals outside Japan. Lancet 1:824-825.
19. Zeng Y, Lan XY, Fang J, Wang PZ, Wang YR, Sui YF, Wang ZT, Hu RJ, Hinuma Y. 1984. HTLV antibody in China. Lancet 1:799-800.
20. Tajima K, Tominaga S, Suchi T. 1984 (in press). Malignant lymphomas in Japan: epidemiological analysis on adult T-cell leukemia/lymphoma. Haematol Oncol 2.
21. Kinoshita K, Hino S, Amagasaki T, Ikeda S, Yamada Y, Suzuyama J, Momita S, Toriya K, Kamihira S, Ichimaru M. 1984. Demonstration of adult T-cell leukemia virus antigen in milk from three sero-positive mothers. Gann 75:103-105.
22. Nakano S, Ichijo M, Hinuma Y, et al. Search for possible routes of vertical and horizontal transmission of adult T-cell leukemia virus. (unpublished)
23. Okochi K, Sato H, Hinuma Y. 1984 (in press). A retrospective study on transmission of adult T-cell leukemia virus by blood transfusion: seroconversion in recipient. Vox Sang.
24. Ichimaru M, Kinoshita K, Kamihira S, Yamada Y, Oyakawa Y, Amagasaki T, Kusano M. 1982. Familial disposition of adult T-cell leukemia and lymphoma. Gann Monogr Cancer Res 28:185-195.
25. Tajima K, Akaza T, Koike K, Hinuma Y, Suchi T, Tominaga S. 1984. HLA antigens and adult T-cell leukemia virus infection: a community based study in the Goto Islands, Japan. Jpn J Clin Oncol 14:347-352.
26. Tajima K, Tominaga S, Suchi T, Fujita K, Oda T, Tochikura T, Hinuma Y. 1984 (in press). Sero-epidemiological analysis of antibody expression against natural infection with ATLV amongst healthy inhabitants in the Goto Islands, Japan: an interim report. In: Manipulation of Host Defence Mechanisms--Fifth Symposium Proceedings. Haddon RA, ed. Excerpta Medica Asia.
27. Miyamoto T, Hino S, Muneshita T. 1983. Seroepidemiological studies of antibody against antigens expressed on adult T-cell leukemia cells in Nagasaki area. In: Leukemia Reviews International. Rich MA, ed. Marcel Dekker, p105.
28. Tajima K, Tominaga S, Shimizu H, Suchi T. 1981. A hypothesis on the etiology of adult T-cell leukemia/lymphoma. Gann Monogr Cancer Res 72:684-691.
29. Tajima K, Fujita K, Tsukidate S, Oda T, Tominaga S, Suchi T, Hinuma Y. 1983. Seroepidemiological studies on the effects of filarial parasites on infestation of adult T-cell leukemia virus in the Goto Islands, Japan. Gann Monogr Cancer Res 74:188-191.
30. Seiki M, Hattori S, Hirayama Y, Yoshida M. 1983. Human adult T-cell leukemia virus: complete nucleotide sequence of the provirus genome integrated in leukemia cell DNA. Proc Natl Acad Sci USA 80:3618-3622.
31. Kinoshita K, Hino S, Amagasaki T, Yamada Y, Kamihira S, Ichimaru M, Munehisa Y, Hinuma Y. 1982. Development of adult T-cell leukemia-lymphoma (ATL) in two anti-ATL-associated antigen-positive healthy adults. Gann Monogr Cancer Res 73:684-685.

IMMUNOHISTOLOGIC TECHNIQUES: THEIR IMPACT IN TUMOR DIAGNOSIS WITH PARTICULAR REFERENCE TO LYMPHOMAS

CLIVE R. TAYLOR, FLORENCE M. HOFMAN, ANDY E. SHERROD, ALAN EPSTEIN

"Tumors are classified like normal tissue on a histologic basis.... The type of cell is the one important element in every tumor. From it the tumor should be named...." -- Mallory (1914)[1]

The diagnosis and classification of lymphoma and leukemia continues to depend upon examination of a cell sample or tissue biopsy. The morphological criteria employed in attaining a diagnosis are based upon clinicopathological correlations compiled by successive generations of pathologists. Although many attempts have been made to define these criteria strictly, they, nonetheless, remain subjective. Their application by different pathologists is greatly influenced by personal bias, educational prejudice, and such circumstantial evidence as the age of the patient, associated signs and symptoms, and the location of the lesion.

Histopathologists and hematologists have, of course, long been cognizant of the subjective nature of morphological diagnosis. Indeed pathologists have adopted a standard strategy for resolving differences of diagnosis (opinion) by soliciting the opinions (diagnoses) of other pathologists until a democratic consensus is achieved. Other pathologists have sought independent means of validating histopathologic criteria. Special histochemical techniques (eg, silver stains, mucin stains, the periodic acid Schiff reaction) were devised and proved useful in some areas of histopathology, although less so with reference to the lymphomas. With the advent of immunohistochemical methods, initially in the form of immunofluorescence techniques, a few investigative pathologists recognized the potential value of a new means of cell identification, which was based upon recognition of the surface and/or cytoplasmic antigenic components of a cell and was independent of morphologic criteria. The implications with reference to tumor pathology are enormous. Traditionally, neoplasms are recognized and classified according to the normal cell type that they most closely resemble.[1] Therefore, if more definitive methods of identifying normal cell types were to become available, the recognition of the corresponding neoplasms would be greatly enhanced.

During early immunohistologic studies of lymphoid tissues and lymphomas, exemplified by the work of Braylan and Rappaport,[2] one critical limitation of the immunofluorescence technique was revealed, namely, the poor morphological resolution that is inherent in the use of ultraviolet light microscopy and cryostat sections. However, the dramatic success of immunofluorescence methods in other areas of pathology (eg, recognition of "autoantibodies" in autoimmune diseases) created an urgent demand for alternate methods of labelling antibodies for immunohistological studies. It was recognized that the use of enzymatic labels had certain advantages, for by the addition of a suitable substrate system it was possible to develop a colored reaction product, visible by light microscopy, at the site of localization of the enzyme-labelled antibody on the tissue section. A number of enzymes were studied for their possible usefulness, including alkaline phosphatase, glucose oxidase, and horseradish peroxidase. From these, horseradish peroxidase emerged as the most useful by virtue of its availability in pure form, its relative stability, and the existence of a wide range of chromogenic substrates for its demonstration in tissues.[3,4]

Initially, immunoperoxidase techniques, in analogy to the corresponding immunofluorescence methods, were applied to cryostat sections. However, it was subsequently realized that within the lymphoid system at least some antigens could be demonstrated in routinely-processed paraffin-embedded material using immunoperoxidase techniques.[5,6] Advantages to using paraffin-embedded material are considerable. Firstly, immunostaining of tissue antigens can be achieved in preparations in which morphologic detail is excellent, equivalent to the usual hematoxylin and eosin-stained paraffin sections upon which pathologists have traditionally based their diagnoses. Secondly, since paraffin-embedded specimens are used, the method is made immediately available to practicing pathologists for diagnostic use in histopathology. By the same token, retrospective studies of material stored as paraffin blocks are possible; studies of relatively rare conditions, that otherwise would require many years of prospective study, can readily be attempted.

Despite these advantages, there is one theoretical drawback, namely that the antigen under study may have been destroyed or denatured to an unknown degree by the processes of fixaton and paraffin embedment, thus compromising the reliability of the method.

IMMUNOPEROXIDASE OR IMMUNOFLUORESCENCE: THE CHOICE

Following initial reports of the demonstration of immunoglobulin antigens in formalin-fixed paraffin-embedded tissues,[5,7] a number of investigators have concentrated their efforts upon comparing immunofluorescence and immunoperoxidase techniques.[8] The principal points of comparison are outlined in Table 1. Review[9] of these publications reveals a consensus that

Table 1. Comparison of Immunoperoxidase with Immunofluorescence Methods for Immunohistologic Diagnosis.

IMMUNOPEROXIDASE		IMMUNOFLUORESCENCE	
Advantages	Disadvantages	Advantages	Disadvantages
Good morphologic detail*	-	-	Poor morphologic detail
Permanent preparation	-	-	Ephemeral staining (label fades)
High sensitivity	-	High sensitivity	-
Examine by light microscopy	-	-	Requirement for fluorescent microscope
May be applied to both frozen & paraffin*	-	-	Usually restricted to frozen sections**
-	Possible Antigen loss*	Good preservation of antigens	-
-	-	-	Background fluorescence

*Morphology excellent in paraffin sections, but some antigens are partially or wholly denatured under these conditions.

**Reactivity may be obtained in fixed paraffin sections, but autofluorescence is severe.

immunoperoxidase and immunofluorescence methods are comparable in terms of specificity and sensitivity. However, these same studies revealed that the effects of fixation can be critical, depending upon the nature of the antigen in question and upon its localization within the tissue under study.[3,10,11] For example, surface immunoglobulin is best demonstrated in unfixed cryostat sections,[8,11] whether by peroxidase or fluorescence; whereas cytoplasmic immunoglobulin can be demonstrated to some degree in both cryostat and fixed paraffin-embedded sections. Indeed, cytoplasmic immunoglobulins are well visualized in the latter situation due to the excellent morphologic detail achieved utilizing the immunoperoxidase technique.

In contemplating any study of tissue antigens, whether for research and investigation or primarily for diagnostic purposes, pathologists should attempt to make a rational assessment of needs and priorities as a means of selecting the optimal immunohistologic procedure. If morphology is of the essence, then the immunoperoxidase technique on paraffin sections is to be preferred; if there is doubt as to antigen preservation or the efficacy of a particular antibody in fixed tissue, then one may need to utilize cryostat sections, recognizing that this incurs some loss of convenience and morphologic resolution.

BASIC TECHNIQUES IN IMMUNOHISTOLOGY

There are several variations of the the immunoperoxidase technique; one or another may be preferred for particular purposes. The principles are schematically represented in Figure 1. The direct conjugate procedure (A) in which the horseradish peroxidase enzyme is directly linked to the primary antibody is used infrequently, for it appears to be less sensitive than the other methods and in addition requires chemical conjugation of the enzyme to the primary antibody which may be in short supply. The indirect conjugate procedure and the peroxidase anti-peroxidase (PAP) method (B) may be used interchangeably; the PAP method[3,4] being more sensitive in some situations, may permit use of the primary antibody at a higher dilution, again an important factor in conserving a precious antibody. Warnke and Levy[12] utilized the biotin-avidin system (C), a method that depends upon the high affinity binding of avidin (conjugated to horseradish peroxidase)

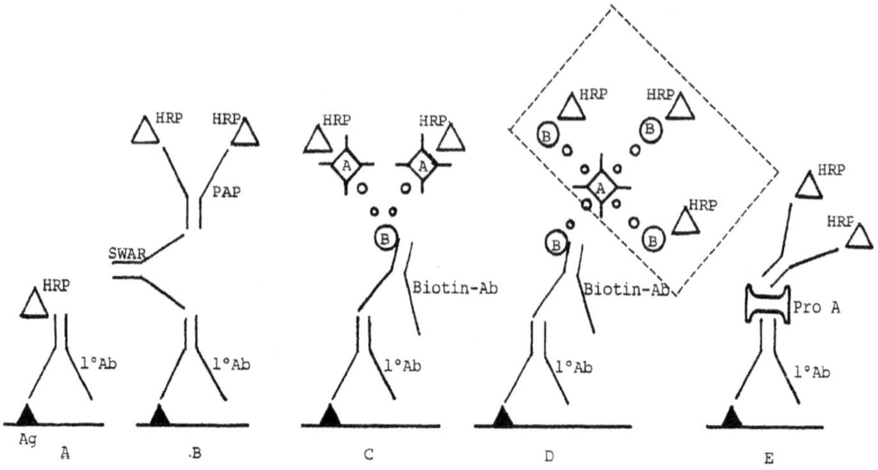

FIGURE 1. Immunoperoxidase Methods: (A) Direct Conjugation, (B) Indirect Conjugation (PAP), (C) Biotin-Avidin, (D) Avidin-Biotin Complex (ABC), (E) Protein A Bridge. Ag=antigen, Ab=antibody, HRP=horseradish peroxidase enzyme, SWAR=swine anti-rabbit antiserum, PAP=peroxidase antiperoxidase complex, B=biotin, A=avidin, Pro A=staphalococcal protein A.

with biotin (conjugated to specific antisera). Warnke and Levy reported that the biotin-avidin system was superior to their enzyme-labelled antibody method, although this has not always been the experience of other investigators comparing these methods. Recent improvements in the biotin-avidin system have increased sensitivity and reduced background staining (D).[13] This, the so-called ABC method, was accomplished by greater purification of the biotinylated antisera and the use of precomplexed avidin-biotin components. The quality of labelling for both paraffin and frozen sections was thereby greatly increased. Finally, staphylococcal protein A has been employed in immunoperoxidase methods (E)[14] to serve as the linking reagent which binds the IgG component of the PAP complex to primary antibody of the IgG class. This gives great versatility in that PAP from one species may be linked to primary antibody of a second species; the method is, however, effective only for particular IgG subclasses. With reasonable organization and strategy, these immunoperoxidase and other enzyme-labelled methods have been introduced into an increasing number of "routine" laboratories throughout Europe and the United States as an adjunct to the standard histologic staining procedures. In these circumstances the immunoperoxidase method is best regarded as a specific, highly versatile special staining technique, comparable in some ways to orthodox histochemical procedures, but having a much higher degree of specificity.

IMMUNOHISTOLOGIC DIAGNOSIS

One obstacle to the more general utilization of immunoenzyme methods for diagnostic purposes was that quality specific primary antisera were available against only a limited range of cellular antigens; hence only a limited number of useful "special stains" were available. Furthermore, the production of such antisera was tedious, requiring purification of antigen, immunization, and affinity absorption of resulting antisera. The advent of the "hybridoma" technique resulted in production of a bewildering array of monoclonal antibodies having specificity against many of the known cell-related antigens or against a range of new cellular antigens directly defined by the newly available antibodies.

The application of these monoclonal antibodies to immunoperoxidase methods opened new areas of investigation in the recognition and classification of tumors in general and lymphomas and leukemias in particular. Monoclonal antibodies identified previously unrecognized lymphoid and monocyte subpopulations.[15] Some of these same antibodies were then used in characterizing lymphoid proliferations.[16] A partial listing of some of the more useful reagents is given in Table 2. A major problem at present is the standardization of monoclonal antibodies from different research and commercial laboratories. This can best be achieved by identifying the membrane antigen to which the antibody binds.[17,18] While this type of information is presently incomplete, studies involving the precipitation and isolation of antigens with monoclonal antibodies have characterized at least some of the target antigens, and attempts are being made to establish correlations between the presence of antigen on the cell,[15] the ontogeny of the cell,[19,20] and the cellular function.[21]

The majority of monoclonal antibodies are currently produced in the mouse system. Since the monoclonal antibody is composed of a single subclass, the characteristics of this subclass must be taken into account when considering a particular labelling technique. For example, if protein A is to be used as the linking

Table 2. Lymphomas--Immunohistologic Recognition and Subclassification

Antibody	Mol wt/ Daltons	Binding Population	Source
A. Antibodies used as screening panel for frozen sections of suspected lymphomas			
*CLA/T29/33	100,000	Pan-leucocyte (common leukocyte antigen)	Dako/HT
Leu 4/OKT8	20,000-30,000	Pan T cells	BD/Ortho
B-1/OKB7	175,000	Pan B cells	Ortho
OKM-1	---	Monocytes, macrophages granulocytes	Ortho
Kappa	23,000	Ig-kappa-bearing cells	Tago
Lambda	23,000	Ig-lambda-bearing cells	Tago
B. Expanded panel for frozen section identification			
Leu 1	67,000	Pan T cell	BD
Leu 5/OKT11	---	E rosette receptor (Pan T cell)	BD/Ortho
Leu 2/OKT8	32,000-43,000	Suppressor/cytotoxic T cells	BD/Ortho
Leu 3/OKT4	55,000	Helper/inducer T cells	BD/Ortho
Leu 7	---	Natural killer cells	BD
OKT6	49,000	Thymocytes	Ortho
T101	67,000	Pan T cells	HT
B-1	30,000	B cells	Coulter
BA-1	65,000	B cells	HT
BA-2	---	Early B cells	HT
B-5	45,000	Mature B cells	UCSD
*LN-1	---	Follicular center B cells	TC
*LN-2	---	B cells/histiocytes	TC
*LN-3	---	Ia-like antigen/B cells/ histiocytes/some T cells	TC
Leu M-1	---	Macrophages/monocytes	BD
CM-1	---	Macrophages/monocytes	UCLA
J-5/CALLA	100,000	Common acute lymphocytic leukemia	Coulter
mu	67,000	IgM-bearing cells	Tago
gamma	53,000	IgG-bearing cells	Tago
delta	70,000	IgD-bearing cells	Tago

These antibodies represent a partial listing of those available: precise specificities, cross reactivities or cross identities of different antibodies from different manufacturers have not been worked out (see text).

*These antibodies also give positive results on paraffin sections.

BD=Becton Dickinson; HT=Hybritech; UCSD=Dr. S. Baird, University of California at San Diego; TC=Techniclone; UCLA=Dr. R. Billing, University of California at Los Angeles.

reagent in the immunoperoxidase method (Figure 1E), then a murine monoclonal antibody of IgG class might be expected to give good results, while an antibody of IgM class would perform poorly. Likewise, if a secondary antibody is to be utilized (in the PAP, ABC or indirect conjugate method), then it is important to select an antibody with strong reactivity for the subclass represented in the primary mouse monoclonal antibody. At the present time no generalization can be made as to which is the optimum procedure for any particular antigen or for any particular antibody. It has become clear that the performance characteristics of different monoclonal antibodies derived from different sources vary dramatically with reference to their applicability to the demonstration of antigens in tissue sections. Thus, when attempting to utilize any new antibody system the investigator is advised that it may be necessary to experiment with one or more of these methods to achieve optimal results.

IMMUNOHISTOLOGIC METHODS APPLIED TO PARAFFIN SECTIONS

Immunoperoxidase methods have been successfully applied to paraffin-embedded sections of normal lymphoid tissue and lymphomas.[5,9,22-26] The techniques employed include the conjugate, peroxidase-antiperoxidase and biotin-avidin methods (Figure 1). Intracellular antigens are often detectable in paraffin-embedded preparations. For example, cytoplasmic immunoglobulin has been demonstrated in plasma cells, immunoblasts and germinal center cells and has been used to study patterns of immunoglobulin staining of lymphoid organs in different developmental and immune states.[5,23,24,27,28] Labelling with anti-kappa and anti-lambda light chains has been important in recognizing monoclonal proliferations of B cells in malignant tissue.[29] However, the great majority of currently available monoclonal antibodies against leucocyte antigens do not give reproducible results in paraffin sections; some notable exceptions are discussed later. The restricted utility of monoclonal antibodies on fixed paraffin sections has given impetus to the use of frozen sections for immunohistologic studies of lymphomas and other tumors.

Various double-staining methods have been developed for the simultaneous demonstration of two antigens in fixed sections.[30] These are of value in precise identification of antigen reactive cells in mixed cell populations within lymphoid tissue. Double immunoperoxidase or immunoperoxidase, alkaline phosphatase, glucose oxidase methods have been described.[23,28,30,31]

IMMUNOHISTOLOGIC METHODS APPLIED TO CRYOSTAT SECTIONS

Experience to date suggests that for the demonstration of membrane antigens, including surface membrane immunoglobulin, best results are obtained using cryostat sections subject to minimal fixation. Surface immunoglobulin is more difficult to detect in sections that are fixed, particularly with formalin,[8,11] This may be due to the destruction (or "masking") of surface membrane proteins during fixation. Surface antigens which are part of the membrane (eg, HLA-Dr or Ia-like antigen) may be exempt from this fate and can be demonstrated in paraffin sections with some antibodies such as LN-3.[26] Though the range of surface antigens detectable in paraffin-embedded sections is limited, this may be as much a function of the lack of availability of the appropriate monoclonal antibody as of antigen destruction per se (vide infra). The detailed morphology of fixed tissues remains an important asset and serves as an incentive for the development of monoclonal antibodies that do give consistent results in fixed paraffin tissues. Studies using both paraffin-embedded and frozen sections in parallel provide the most complete picture of the cellular components of lymphoid tissue.

The methods using frozen material, as advocated by Tubbs,[32] Warnke and Levy[12] and Janossy[33] are basically similar. Briefly, small (10mm) blocks of tissue are taken fresh from the biopsy, quick-frozen in either isopentane and dry ice or liquid nitrogen directly. The cut sections are fixed in cold acetone for periods varying from 10 seconds to 20 minutes. In essence, the longer the period of acetone fixation, the better the resulting morphologic detail, but the higher the probability of significant loss of antigenicity. Thus some compromise should be reached in deciding the optimal duration of fixation; the time selected will not necessarily be the same for different membrane antigens. For example, surface immunoglobulin is readily demonstrable after 20 minutes in acetone; whereas detection of some of the T cell surface antigens may be seriously compromised after more than 10 minutes in acetone. This may be related to the chemical composition of the antigen and its location in the membrane. Many T cell antigens are glycoproteins and extremely sensitive to formaldehyde and glutaraldehyde treatment. Their antigenic properties, however, are retained after a 10 second exposure to acetone; progressive loss of antigenicity then appears to occur. Serologically defined antigens may be located intracellularly or as part of the membrane structure. The antigenic determinants, such as the HLA-Dr (Ia-like) antigens, are integrated into the membrane, while the T-cell antigens appear to be more loosely attached to the outside of the lipid bilayer.[34] Both the cellular location of the antigen and its structure appear to influence the extent to which it resists fixation and processing.

Following the preparation of the acetone-fixed cryostat sections, either immunofluorescence or immunoperoxidase techniques may be employed for visualization of the antigen. If detailed morphological studies are envisaged, in order to examine critically the types of cells that show positive or negative staining for any particular antigen, then there is no substitute for utilizing the immunoperoxidase method with one or other of the more common nuclear counterstains, such as hematoxylin.

STAINING OF CELL SUSPENSIONS, CYTOCENTRIFUGE AND IMPRINT PREPARATIONS

Both immunofluorescence and immunoperoxidase methods can be applied to labelling of surface antigens on viable cell suspensions. Immunofluorescence has been used widely for this purpose in enumerating surface immunoglobulin-bearing cells.[35] Cell suspensions provide a way to quantitate the number of labelled cells and thus provide some objectivity. With the advent of monoclonal antibodies distinguishing subpopulations of lymphocytes, diseases like leukemias have been subclassified according to immunologic markers; the information provided has been successfully used in determining differential prognosis and treatment.[16,36-41]

The procedure for labelling cells in suspension must take into account the problems of cell viability and modulation of surface antigens. Cells are isolated from fresh material (eg, lymph node biopsies or peripheral blood). To obtain cells from tissue, the specimen is gently teased in phosphate-buffered saline containing bovine serum albumin or fetal calf serum and sodium azide. The cells are released into the medium during this process. To recover cells from peripheral blood, whole blood is layered on a Ficoll-Hypaque density gradient; the lymphocytes are isolated from the interface as a partially purified population. The cells recovered from the tissue or whole blood must be counted and examined for viability, usually using the trypan blue dye exclusion method, since dead cells will alter the cell count due to nonspecific intracellular staining in both immunofluorescence and immunoperoxidase techniques. Bovine serum albumin in the phosphate-buffered saline solution appears to improve viability during the preparation and isolation procedure. Capping and involution of surface antigens can be eliminated by the use to the metabolic inhibitor, sodium azide. At low concentrations of this substance (0.02%), there is no effect on viability. Alternatively, the staining procedure can be performed at 4C; at this temperature the membrane antigens are also stabilized.

Fluorescein-labelled viable cells in suspension may be examined (by manual microscopy or by automated cytofluorometry),[42] a significant advantage when equipment is available. The principal limitation of all the labelling techniques is the threshold density of antigen for visualization. Fluorescence-activated cell analyses have increased the sensitivity of the immunofluorescence technique; this apparatus can now detect as few as 3,000 fluorescent molecules per cell. The fluorescence-activated cell sorters are currently being used as research tools to separate the labelled from non-labelled cells, allowing investigators to identify the functional properties of the stained cells, be they normal or malignant sub-populations. The same panel of antibodies that is utilized in cytofluorometric analysis may be used to stain cryostat sections in order to visualize the cell populations and their interrelationships in situ.

Using a panel of monoclonal antibodies which recognize sub-populations of T cells, it has been shown that many lymphocytes bear more than one of the corresponding surface antigens.[19,20] The presence of a particular membrane antigen may not be unique to a cell series but may simply signify a developmental stage of the cell.[20] This has been clearly delineated for T cell maturation. In man, the T11 antigen is expressed on the majority of early fetal thymocytes, predominantly in the cortex, the less mature region of the thymus. In contrast, the T6 antigen appears later in this organ, but is lost before the T cell enters into the peripheral blood cell pool. Certain antigens that formerly were thought to be lineage restricted (eg, OKT6) turn out, on further investigation, to be present on unrelated cell types (OKT6 in Langerhans cells) further complicating the use of these reagents as "special stains" for particular cell types. The presence of still other antigens may reflect the state of activation of the cell or the stage of cell cycle. A quiescent T cell does not possess the Dr antigen; however, upon stimulation, this antigen becomes detectable.[43,44]

As an alternative to cytofluorometry, which requires expensive equipment, cytocentrifuge preparations are easily prepared and provide a good way of visualizing the cytologic features of the tissue cell suspension or peripheral blood. Immunoperoxidase techniques can be used to identify subpopulations using monoclonal antibodies or specific conventional antisera. The cytocentrifuge preparations are made using cells resuspended in phosphate-buffered saline with either fetal calf serum or bovine serum albumin; serum promotes adherence of the cells to the slide. These cytocentrifuge preparations are then air dried and may be stored at room temperature for several weeks. The staining procedure for immunoperoxidase is similar to the technique described for paraffin sections or blood films.[45] The cytocentrifuge preparations are exposed to H_2O_2 in methanol, which fixes the cells and eliminates endogenous peroxidase activity. The specimens are then exposed to the primary antibody followed by labelling reagents (PAP, ABC or conjugate systems). A 10 second fixation with acetone may be utilized before application of the primary antibody. For nuclear detail the slides are counterstained with hematoxylin. Immunoperoxidase has the advantage of simultaneously exhibiting staining and excellent morphologic detail under the light microscope.

Double-labelling immunoenzyme techniques are particularly useful in cytocentrifuge preparations, permitting visualization of two antigens in single cells simultaneously. Both surface and cytoplasmic antigens can be demonstrated by suitable manipulation of the staining sequence; viable cells in suspension are first labelled for a particular surface antigen; various substrates can be used to visualize these surface determinants (ie, diaminobenzidine--brown; amino-ethyl carbazole--red). These labelled cells can then be cytocentrifuged, fixed and stained for cytoplasmic antigens using the contrasting grey reaction product of 4-chloro-1-naphthol[46] or using an alkaline phosphatase or glucose oxidase system.

APPROACH TO DIAGNOSIS OF LYMPHOMA BY IMMUNOHISTOLOGY

A prerequisite for effective immunohistologic studies of lymphomas, and other tumors, is active involvement of the clinicians and surgeons. Ideally, every biopsy or resection of a tumor, or suspected tumor, should be submitted immediately to the pathologist in a fresh unfixed state. The pathologist should slice and inspect the tissue, selecting material for fixation and embedding as part of the "routine diagnostic" procedure, but reserving other tissue for possible immunohistologic studies as described below. Fixation, if in formalin, should be for the minimum time consistent with good morphology; fresh buffered formalin should be used. Processing and embedment should be carefully controlled, particularly the temperature of the paraffin bath. Additional tissue should be fixed in B5, since many antigens show superior survival when fixed in this way. Finally, tissue should be frozen and "banked." Ideally, small segments of tissue should be frozen and stored in liquid nitrogen or a -70C freezer. Failing that, small blocks of tissue held at -30C in the cryostat cabinet serve as a short-term resource for performance of frozen section immunohistology if the need for such studies becomes apparent after examining the H&E sections.

When the H&E sections are examined, the pathologist may be confident of the diagnosis, electing to issue a report without additional studies. If there is doubt as to the nature or classification of the lesion, then "special stains" may be ordered; these may include immunohistochemical stains. Practically, a first step is to perform whatever stains may appear relevant and feasible on paraffin sections (formalin or B5 fixed) (Table 3). Antibodies that are reproducibly effective include antibody to common leucocyte antigen (CLA) (not all anti-CLA antibodies work in paraffin sections), Ia-like (HLA-Dr) antigen (eg, LN-3,[26] see Table 2), LN-2[25] (B cells and histiocytes), LN-1[25] (follicular center B cells), Leu-M1 (some histiocytes) and antibodies versus immunoglobulin

Table 3. Applications of Immunohistologic Methods in Hematopathology--Paraffin Sections*

Immunoglobulin

1. Distinction of reactive B cell proliferations from B cell neoplasia ("monoclonal")
   a. Myeloma--benign monoclonal gammopathy--reactive plasmacytosis
   b. Plasmacytoid lymphocytic lymphoma/plasmacytoma--chronic reactive lymphadenitis
   c. Follicular center cell lymphoma (some cases)--reactive follicular hyperplasia
   d. B cell immunoblastic sarcoma--reactive immunoblastic proliferations
2. Subclassification of lymphomas
   a. Recognition of B cell tumors by Ig content
   b. Subclassification of B cell tumors
3. Recognition of anaplastic tumor as B cell in origin according to content of monoclonal Ig (distinction of B-immunoblastic sarcoma from carcinoma, melanoma, etc)
4. Recognition of morphologically unusual tumors as B cell in origin (eg, "signet ring cell" lymphoma)

J Chain--Recognition of B cell nature of normal or neoplastic cells

Lysozyme

1. Histiocytic marker in reactive and neoplastic proliferations
2. Marker of primary granule formation in myeloid maturation
3. Distinction of granulocytic sarcoma from other "anaplastic" tumors
4. Rapid identification of numbers of granulocytes in marrow (marrow granulocyte reserve)

Alpha-l-antitrypsin, chymotrypsin--Aid to recognition of reactive and neoplastic histiocytes

Lactoferrin

1. Marker of secondary granule formation in meyloid maturation
2. Aid to assessment of mature granulocytes in marrow

Hemoglobin A and F

1. Distinction of erythroid precursors from lymphoid cells
2. Rapid and specific identification of marrow erythroid reserve, from stage of hemoglobin synthesis
3. Assessment of extent of HBF production in marrow in hemolytic diseases

LN-1--Recognition of follicular center cell lymphomas and normal counterparts

LN-2--Recognition of B cell and histiocytic tumors and normal counterparts; positivity in many Reed-Sternberg cells

LN-3--Recognition of B cell and histiocytic tumors

CLA (common leucocyte antigen)--Recognition of leucocyte tumors (all lymphomas)

---

*Some antigens (eg, immunoglobulins) are better visualized following trypsin digestion.[10]

light and heavy chains.

If the differential diagnosis extends beyond lymphoma to undifferentiated carcinoma, melanoma, germ cell tumor or various sarcomas, then certain other reagents may be useful in excluding lymphoma as a possibility (eg, positivity for keratin in tumor cells excluding lymphoma) (Table 4).

The precision of diagnosis by such methods is sometimes remarkable, as in the use of LN-1 antibody. Lymphoid cells reactive with this antibody are exclusively follicular center cells, including both normal cells and their malignant counterparts. Thus reactive follicles are positive as are follicular center cell lymphomas (both follicular and diffuse).[25,26,47] Interestingly, the Reed-Sternberg cell variants of nodular lymphocyte predominant Hodgkin's disease also show positivity with LN-1,[49] suggesting that this disease may be derived from (or related to) the follicular center cell lymphomas (ie, that this subset of Hodgkin's disease is a B cell neoplasm--Reed-Sternberg cells of the other subclasses of Hodgkin's disease are nonreactive with this antibody).

A BEWILDERING ARRAY OF REAGENTS

Monoclonal antibodies have served as a tremendous stimulus to immunohistologic research. Now, however, the immunohistologist is in danger of drowning in a sea of plenty. Ortho Diagnostics, one of the first major commercial groups to release leucocyte-related monoclonal antibodies, now lists 13 different antibodies; Becton Dickinson lists 25, Hybritech lists six others and there are at least a dozen other suppliers with another 50 or so antibodies. Clearly many of these antibodies are the same (ie, although derived from a separate fusion they recognize the same antigen). Equally, however, others differ in major or minor ways, or in ways so subtle that we cannot recognize the differences as yet. This problem is exemplifed by reference to Table 2. This list is far from comprehensive, including only those reagents for which we have developed some preference based on personal experience. It is possible for other investigators to conduct exhaustive studies with panels of 30 or more antibodies that include only a few of those listed in Table 2.[50,51]

This diversity poses a problem for the hematopathologist seeking diagnostic utility. It has become impossible to remember

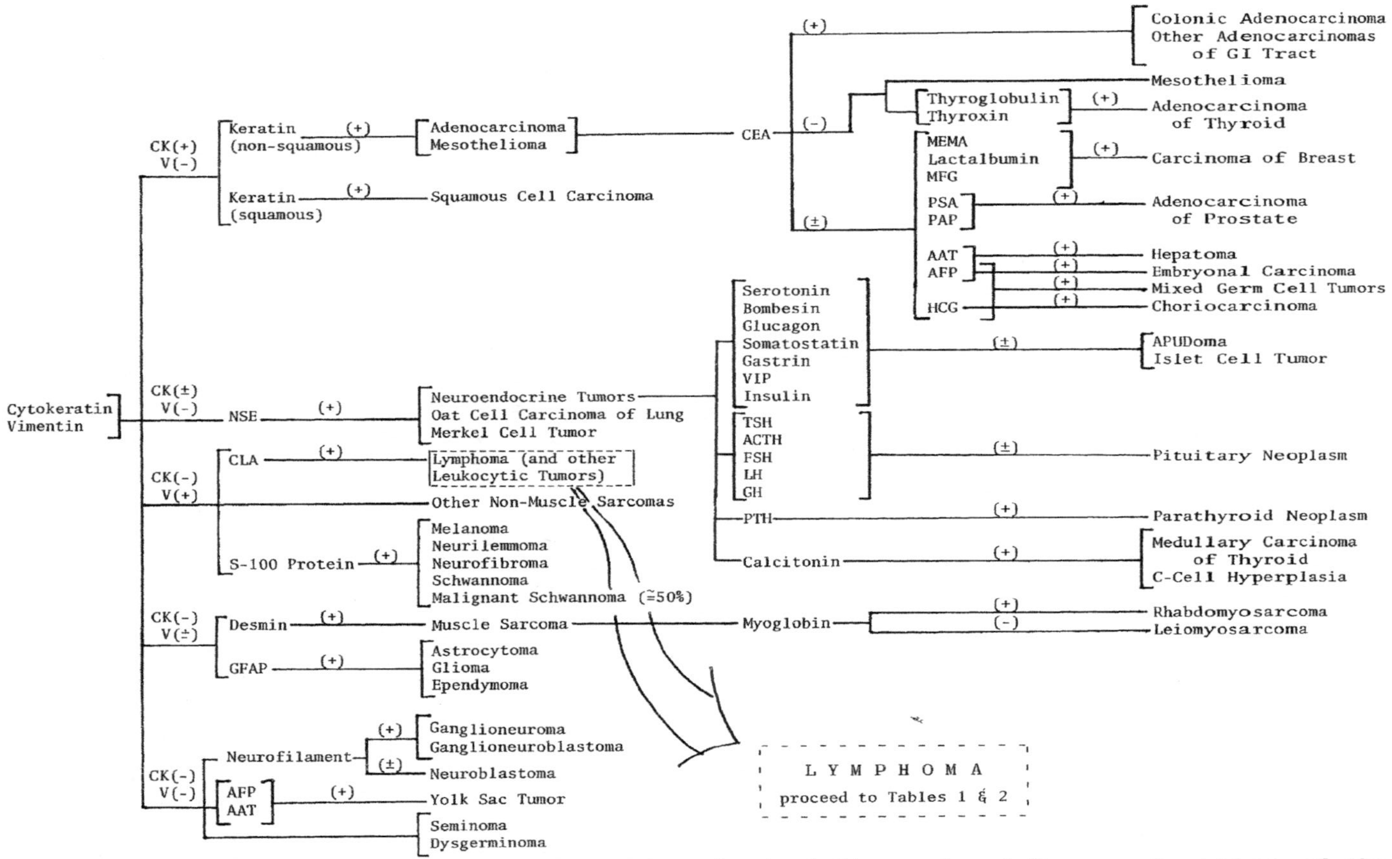

FIGURE 4. Diagnostic Algorithm for Immunohistochemical Diagnosis of Tumors: Position of the Lymphomas in an Immunologic Scheme for Tumor Recognition (modified from reference 47).

the spectrum of reactivity (versus normal and neoplastic cells) of the antibodies produced by a single manufacturer, let alone remembering how these correspond (or fail to correspond) to antibodies from a different source. This problem is compounded by the lack of good data concerning the clinical utility of the information provided by phenotyping studies of lymphomas. Dr. Bharat Nathwani (personal communication) has drawn an apt parallel between the potential for confusion invoked by the immunologic classification of lymphomas (by monoclonal antibodies) and the frenzy produced by the so-called functional (immunologic in concept) classifications of the non-Hodgkin lymphomas that the morphologists championed 10 years ago. The latter conflict still is not resolved.

There is nonetheless cause for optimism. Carefully controlled studies of the utility of these reagents are needed, with cross correlations of different antibodies from differing sources. For simplicity, an individual pathologist may wish to patronize a single source as far as is possible, turning to "specialty houses" when a unique reagent is required (eg, LN-1 for follicular center B cells from Techniclone, Santa Ana, California).

INTERPRETATION

In our quest for improvement in diagnosis and our thirst for individual academic advancement, we are readily beguiled by the easy publications that monoclonal antibodies offer: a new antibody, a new pattern of reactivity, a new paper. As investigators we would do well to remember Goethe's advice:

"Science has been seriously retarded by the study of what is not worth knowing and of what is not knowable."--von Goethe (1749-1832)

The analysis of the data must be made in terms of the number of positive versus negative cells; however, the definition of positivity is critical, particularly whether a positive reaction with a specific monoclonal antibody is observed in malignant cells, in normal cells, or in both. The intensity of the staining must be noted; this intensity may vary with the antibody titer, or the density of antigen per cell. Changes in the number or location of antigenic sites in normal and malignant cells are not well understood. The location of labelled cells throughout the tissue preparation (eg, diffuse or localized) is also an important parameter in correlating existing systems of lymphoma classification with the new immunological methods. Learning how to perform and interpret immunohistologic stains does require a commitment of time and resources; however, in view of the precision of cell and tumor recognition that the method offers, there seems little doubt such a commitment is both necessary and justified.

"There is a 17 year span between consensus in the literature on the utility of a new test and its appropriate use by virtually all (concerned) physicians." --Johnson, 1983[52]

Finally, experience gleaned from the introduction of other basic techniques into "routine diagnostic practice" suggests that, given the commitment and resources, there will still be a lag period before full application of immunohistologic techniques to tumor diagnosis. With the introduction of immunoperoxidase techniques primarily for routine diagnosis having occurred early in the 1970's, it may be expected that the next few years will see this technique approach its full potential among surgical pathologists engaged in the diagnosis of tumors.

REFERENCES

1. Mallory FBP. 1914. In: The Princples of Pathologic Histology. Philadelphia, WB Saunders Co, p 333.
2. Braylan RC, Rappaport H. 1973. Tissue immunoglobulins in nodular lymphomas as compared with reactive follicular hyperplasias. Blood 42:579-589.
3. Sternberger LA. 1979. Immunochemistry, 2nd ed. New York, John Wiley & Sons Inc, pp 104-169.
4. Taylor CR. 1978. Immunoperoxidase techniques: theoretical and practical aspects. Arch Pathol Lab Med 102:113-121.
5. Taylor CR. 1974. The nature of Reed-Sternberg cells and other malignant cells. Lancet 2:802-807.
6. Burns J, Hambridge M, Taylor CR. 1974. Intracellular immunoglobulins: A comparative study on three standard tissue processing methods using horseradish peroxidase and fluorochrome conjugates. J Clin Pathol 27:548.
7. Taylor CR, Burns J. 1974. The demonstration of plasma cells and other immunoglobulin containing cells in formalin-fixed, paraffin-embedded tissues using peroxidase labelled antibody. J Clin Pathol 27:548-557.
8. Curran RC, Gregory J. 1978. Demonstration of immunoglobulin in cryostat and paraffin sections of human tonsil by immunofluorescence and immunoperoxidase techniques. J Clin Pathol 31:974-983.
9. Taylor CR. 1980. Immunohistologic studies of lymphoma: past, present and future. J Histochem Cytochem 28:777-787.
10. DeLellis RA. 1981. Diagnostic Immunohistochemistry. New York,

Masson.
11. Warnke R. 1979. Alteration of immunoglobulin-bearing lymphoma cells by fixation. J Histochem Cytochem 27:1195-1196.
12. Warnke R, Levy R. 1980. Detection of T and B cell antigens with hybridoma monoclonal antibodies: a biotin-avidin-horseradish peroxidase method. J HistochemCytochem 28:771-776.
13. Hsu SM, Raine L, Fanger H. 1981. The use of avidin-biotin-peroxidase complex (ABC) in immunoperoxidase techniques: a comparison between ABC and unlabeled antibody (PAP) procedures. J Histochem Cytochem 29:577-580.
14. Notani GW, Parsons JA, Erlandsen SL. 1979. Versatility of Staphylococcus aureus Protein A in immunochemistry. J Histochem Cytochem 27:1438-1444.
15. Kung PC, Goldstein G, Reinherz EL, Schlossman SF. 1979. Monoclonal antibodies defining distinctive human T cell surface antigens. Science 206:347-349.
16. Aisenberg AC. 1981. Cell-surface markers in lymphoproliferative disease. N Engl J Med 304:331-336.
17. Andersson LC, Gahmberg CG, Nilsson K, Wigzell H. 1977. Surface glycoprotein patterns of normal and malignant human lymphoid cells: T cells, T blasts and leukemic T cell lines. Int J Cancer 20:702-707.
18. Royston I, Majda JA, Baird SM, Meserve BL, Griffiths JC. 1980. Human T cell antigens defined by monoclonal antibodies: the 65,000 dalton antigen of T cells (T65) is also found on chronic lymphocytic leukemia cells bearing surface immunoglobulin. J Immunol 125:725-731.
19. Bhan AK, Reinherz EL, Poppema S, McCluskey RT, Schlossman SF. 1980. Location of T cell and major histocompatibility complex antigens in the human thymus. J Exp Med 152:771-782.
20. Janossy G, Tidmann N, Papageorgiou ES, Kung PC, Goldstein G. 1981. Distribution of T lymphocyte subsets in the human bone marrow and thymus: an analysis with monoclonal antibodies. J Immunol 126:1608-1613.
21. Reinherz EL, Kung PC, Goldstein G, Schlossman SF. 1979. Separation of functional subsets of human T cells by monoclonal antibody. Proc Natl Acad Science USA 76:4061-4065.
22. Isaacson P, Wright DH, Judd MA, Jones DB, Payne SV. 1980. The nature of the immunoglobulin-containing cells in malignant lymphoma: an immunoperoxidase study. J Histochem Cytochem 28:761-770.
23. Taylor CR. 1976. An immunohistological study of follicular lymphoma, reticulum cell sarcoma and Hodgkin's disease. Eur J Cancer 12:61-75.
24. Taylor CR. 1978. Immunocytochemical methods in the study of lymphoma and related conditions. J Histochem Cytochem 26:496-512.
25. Epstein AL, Marder RJ, Winter J, Fox RI. 1984. Two new monoclonal antibodies (LN-1, LN-2) reactive in B5 fixed paraffin embedded tissues with follicular center and mantle zone human B lymphocytes and derived tumors. J Immunol 133:1028-1036.
26. Marder RJ, Variakojis D, Silver J, Epstein AL. 1985 (in press). Immunohistochemical analysis of human lymphomas with monoclonal antibodies to B-cell and Ia antigens reactive in paraffin sections. Lab Invest.
27. Stein H, Bank A, Tolksdorf G, Rodt H, Gerdes J. 1980. Immunohistologic analysis of the organization of normal lymphoid tissue and non-Hodgkin's lymphomas. J Histochem Cytochem 28:746-760.

28. Taylor CR, Mason DY. 1974. Immunohistological detection of intracellular immunoglobulin in formalin-paraffin sections from multiple myeloma using the immunoperoxidase technique. Clin Exp Immunol 18:417-429.
29. Levy R, Warnke R, Dorfman RF, Haimovich J. 1977. The monoclonality of human B-cell lymphomas. J Exp Med 145:1014-1028.
30. Falini B, De Solas I, Halverson C, Parker JW, Taylor CR. 1982. A new two-stage double immunoenzymatic method for labeling of intracellular antigens in paraffin-embedded tissues. J Histochem Cytochem 30:21-26.
31. Mason DY, Sammons R. 1978. Alkaline phosphatase and peroxidase for double immunoenzymatic labelling of cellular constituents. J Clin Pathol 31:454-460.
32. Tubbs RR, Sheibani K, Sebek BA, Weiss RA. 1980. Immunohistochemistry versus immunofluorescence for non-Hodgkin lymphomas. Am J Clin Pathol 73:144-145.
33. Janossy G, Thomas JA, Habeshaw JA. 1980. Immunofluorescence analysis of normal and malignant lymphoid tissues with selected combination of antisera. J Histochem Cytochem 28:1207-1214.
34. Walsh FS, Crumpton MJ. 1977. Orientation of cell-surface antigens in the lipid bilayer of lymphocyte plasma membranes. Nature 269:307-311.
35. Raff MC, Steinberg M, Taylor RB. 1970. Immunoglobulin determinants on the mouse lymphoid cells. Nature 225:553-554.
36. Borella L, Sen L, Casper JT. 1977. Acute lymphoblastic leukemia (ALL) antigens detected with antisera to E-rosette-forming ALL blasts. J Immunol 118:309-315.
37. Brouet JC, Seligmann M. 1978. The immunological classification of acute lymphoblastic leukemias. Cancer 42:817-827.
38. Greaves MF, Brown G, Rapson NT, Lister TA. 1975. Antisera to acute lymphoblastic leukemia cells. Clin Immunol Immunopathol 4:67-84.
39. Pesando JM, Ritz J, Lazarus H, Costello SB, Sallan S, Schlossman SF. 1979. Leukemia-associated antigens in ALL. Blood 54:1240-1248.
40. Reinherz EL, Nadler LM, Sallan SE, Schlossman SF. 1979. Subset derivation of T-cell acute lymphoblastic leukemia in man. J Clin Invest 64:392-397.
41. Tsukimoto I, Wong KY, Lampkin BC. 1976. Surface markers and prognostic factors in acute lymphoblastic leukemia. N Engl J Med 294:245-248.
42. Herzenberg LA, Herzenberg LA. 1978. Analysis and separation using the fluorescence activated cell sorter (FACS). In: Handbook of Experimental Immunology, 3rd ed, Weir DM (Ed). Oxford, Blackwell, pp 99-109.
43. Fu SM, Chiorazzi N, Wang CY, et al. 1978. Ia-bearing T lymphocytes in man: their identification and role in the generation of allogeneic helper activity. J Exp Med 148:1423-1427.
44. Reinherz EL, Kung PC, Pesando JM, Ritz J, Goldstein G, Schlossman SF. 1979. Ia determinants on human T cell subsets defined by monoclonal antibody: activation stimuli required for expression. J Exp Med 150:1472-1482.
45. Mason DY, Farrell C, Taylor CR. 1975. The detection of intracellular antigens in human leucocytes by immunoperoxidase staining. Br J Haematol 31:361-370.
46. Hofman FM, Billing RJ, Parker JW, Taylor CR. 1982. Cytoplasmic as opposed to surface Ia antigens expressed on human

peripheral blood lymphocytes and monocytes. Clin Exp Immunol 49:355-363.
47. Sherrod A, Taylor CR. 1985 (in press). Non-lymphocyte tumor markers in tissues. In: Manual of Clinical Immunology. American Society of Microbiology.
48. Okon E, Felder B, Epstein A, et al. 1985 (in press). Monoclonal antibodies reactive with B lymphocytes and histiocytes in paraffin sections. Cancer.
49. Sherrod AE, Felder B, Levy N, Epstein A, Marder R, Lukes RJ, Taylor CR. 1985 (submitted). Immunohistologic identification of phenotypic antigens associated with Hodgkin and Reed-Sternberg cells: a paraffin section study.
50. Pallesen G, Beverley PCL, Lane EB, Madsen M, Mason DY, Stein H. 1984. Nature of non-B, non-T lymphomas: an immunohistological study on frozen tissues using monoclonal antibodies. J Clin Pathol 37:911-918.
51. Stein H, Gatter KC, Heryet A, Mason DY. 1984. Freeze-dried paraffin-embedded human tissue for antigen labelling with monoclonal antibodies. Lancet 2:71.
52. Johnson JL. 1983. Growing leaner: a cost cutting strategy. 1983. Med Lab Observ 15:89-99.

SEROLOGIC APPROACHES TO TUMOR DIAGNOSIS

HANS HANSEN

INTRODUCTION

Extensive efforts have been expended in the area of serological detection to tumor diagnosis. Basically this area of study has been evaluated using three distinct immunologic approaches. The first encompasses tests which detect immune responses to tumor "putative" specific antigens; in the case of human cancer little success has been achieved. A closely related endeavor has been made to develop assays which measure impairment of the immune response caused by tumor products, ie, an attempt to serologically measure the delayed hypersensitivity defect. Again, equivalent blood assays to measure this immune parameter have not found general acceptance in the clinical laboratory. Noteworthy success has been achieved by a third approach, the development of assays which detect antigens associated with neoplasms, termed tumor-associated antigens (TAAs). A major shortcoming of these assays is that the TAAs presently identified demonstrate cross reactivity with normal adult tissue counterparts, as well as share inherent properties with embryonic or fetal tissues, thereby negating tumor specificity.

The objectives of this presentation are two-fold. First, to review the assays for tumor-associated antigens presently used in clinical laboratories, and secondly, to discuss the effects of cancer on the immune system with particular emphasis on altered cellular immune responses and autoimmune phenomena.

LEUKEMIA/LYMPHOMA-ASSOCIATED ANTIGENS

The application of heterologous antisera and monoclonal antibodies have proven to be powerful tools in characterizing and diagnosing lymphoid neoplasms. Table 1 lists some of the reagents which are used routinely to identify those antigens found on B and T lymphocytes.

Table 1. Antibodies to lymphocyte surface antigens useful for serological diagnosis of leukemias and lymphomas.

Antibody	Reference	
anti-SIg	Aisenberg & Wilkes	(1981)[1]
anti-kappa	Minowada et al	(1982)[2]
anti-lambda	Minowada et al	(1982)[2]
OKT1	Knowles et al	(1983)[3]
OKT3	Greaves et al	(1982)[4]
OKT4	Janossy et al	(1982)[5]
OKT8	Greaves et al	(1981)[6]
OKT9	Greaves et al	(1981)[7]
OKT10	Greaves et al	(1981)[7]
OKT11	Greaves et al	(1981)[8]
OKB2	Knowles et al	(1984)[9]
OKB7	Knowles et al	(1984)[9]
anti-cALLa	Ritz et al	(1980)[10]
anti-TdT	Mertelsman et al	(1980)[11]
anti-Cmu	Foon et al	(1982)[12]
anti-Dr	Brodsky et al	(1979)[13]

It is now clear that lymphoid neoplasms can be distinguished phenotypically with monoclonal antibodies, making it possible to relate these malignancies with precise stages of cell differentation. These classifications may be valuable in determining potential therapeutic approaches, classifying leukemias and lymphomas, and monitoring the effects of therapy.

Because these proteins are simply differentiation antigens present on normal lymphocytes, their usefulness as tumor-specific markers is limited. Although a few serum lymphoid TAA assays have been developed, they have not found widespread clinical utility.

CARCINOMA TUMOR-ASSOCIATED ANTIGENS

Carcinoma TAAs are also cell differentiation antigens but are present in serum, unlike lymphoma/leukemia TAAs which are primarily cell bound. Many carcinoma TAAs are present on molecules that are secreted as part of the epithelial cell glycocalyx, which for all practical purposes is outside the body. As a carcinoma arises, the epithelial cells turn into the underlying basement membrane with the concomitant secretion of many components of the glycocalyx. As a result, secreted glycoproteins are released inside the body, thereby gaining access to the vascular system. Excess levels in the circulation makes quantitation of these antigens a useful assay. In tissues, these antigens can be located due to their presence in inappropriate sites as well as in excessive quantities.

Numerous carcinoma TAAs have been identified, such as carcinoembryonic antigen (CEA),[14] alpha-fetoprotein (AFP),[15] human chorionic gonadotropin hormon (HCG),[16] prostatic acid phosphatase (PAP),[17] gross cystic disease protein (GCDP),[18] CA 19-9,[19] CA 125,[20] and CSAp[21] and are now being evaluated for clinical usefulness. CEA, AFP, HCG, and PAP basically are used to: (1) confirm the presence of tumor in patients with disease symptoms, (2) monitor the effectiveness of therapy, (3) detect tumor reoccurrence after therapy, and (4) develop an accurate prognosis.[22-24] For example, colorectal carcinoma, the primary tumor of the gastrointestinal tract, consists of one dominant phenotype (90%) which produces CEA. This markedly enhances the value of CEA as an adjunctive diagnostic aid for use in patients presenting symptoms compatible with this neoplasm. HCG has also been used successfully in trophoblastic disease.[25] Monitoring the level of HCG titers is presently being used to predict disease as well as to develop therapy.

In contrast, carcinomas of the lung and breast consist of numerous histological phenotypes, and the identification of a common organ TAA may be an unrealistic goal. However, it is encouraging that a breast carcinoma "CEA-like" equivalent has been described recently, even though breast carcinoma consists of multiple phenotypic histotypes.[26]

Table 2 depicts the number of new cancer cases observed in the United States each year and the percentage of each major organ type of carcinoma which produce significant elevated serum levels of TAAs. The considerably greater number of carcinoma patients which are candidates for CEA monitoring is apparent.

A rapidly expanding amount of research is now being directed toward developing monoclonal antibodies to epithelial-derived tumors. This offers a promising approach and will hopefully aid in further characterizing the nature and specificity of tumor-associated antigens.

EFFECTS OF CANCER ON THE IMMUNE RESPONSE

Numerous immunologic phenomena occur during neoplastic growth. One of the most obvious effects of neoplasia on the immune system is decreased immune competence as demonstrated by delayed type hypersensitivity skin testing.[27] The types of assays to detect

Table 2. Usefulness of cancer markers related to disease sites

Carcinoma Organ site	CEA %	AFP %	PAP %	GCDP %	No Marker	New cases per year
Digestive	80	3	-	-	17	200,000
Genital	8	7*	48	-	37	156,000
Lung	66	-	-	-	34	143,000
Breast	33	-	-	33	34	113,000
Bladder/Kidney	-	-	-	-	100	55,000

*AFP and HCG combined account for 7% of those identified.

this impairment include: lymphocyte functions such as proliferation responses to mitogens and antigens or generation of cytotoxic lymphocytes; antibody production; impairment of NK cell activity and ADCC activity, etc. Although many patients with metastatic cancer have demonstrated impairment of delayed hypersensitivity, as detected by skin testing, decreased lymphocyte proliferation and decreased NK cell activity and ADCC activity, test results in patients as well as normal individuals tend to fluctuate considerably.[28-30] To make these assays suitable for large-scale clinical application, it would be necessary to standardize the assays and reduce the variability of these tests. To date, the development of a simple, reproducible, serological assay to quantitate depression of immune competence has not been achieved.

TUMOR-SPECIFIC ANTIGENS

Hundreds of claims have been made that tumor-specific antigens have been detected using assays which quantitate the effector cells of ADCC disease syndromes, inflammatory syndromes, delayed hypersensitivity syndromes or cytotoxic T-lymphocyte syndromes. Over the years many of the assays have been evaluated, and unfortunately, the end results have been equivocal at best. Assays claimed to detect tumor-specific antigens and antibodies in sera have also failed in blind testing.

AUTOIMMUNE RESPONSES TO CANCER ANTIGENS

One area that needs further evaluation is the formation of autoantibodies and immune complexes in response to a tumor antigen. The development of autoantibodies occurs in inflammatory disease syndromes such as rheumatoid arthritis and SLE and in membrane receptor-blocking syndromes such as myasthenia gravis and thyrotoxicosis. In the former, immune complexes are formed, and in the latter anti-receptor antibodies are formed. Until recently, assays for circulating immune complexes have suffered from the lack of standardization of both reagents and procedure. Recently these problems have been remedied with the development of assays employing monoclonal antibodies to detect both Clq-Ig and C3d-Ig.[31] Commercial availability of these assays should allow follow up of studies such as those of Dent et al, who have found increased levels of Clq-binding activity in patients with lung cancer and have shown that elevated levels correlate with disease extent and with impaired survival.[32]

In addition, advances in molecular biology are providing powerful new tools to search for oncogene products. Hopefully, application of these new tools will provide leads for the development of serological assays that are more specific and sensitive indicators of neoplastic growth.

REFERENCES

1. Aisenberg AC, Wilkes BM. 1980. Unusual human lymphoma phenotype defined by monoclonal antibody. J Exp Med 152:1126-1131.
2. Minowada J, Sagawa K, Trowbridge IS, Kung PC, Goldstein G. 1982. Marker profiles of 55 human leukemia-lymphoma cell lines. In: Malignant Lymphomas: Etiology, Immunology, Pathology and Treatment, Rosenberg SA, Kaplan HS, eds. New York, Academic Press, pp 53-74.
3. Knowles DM, Halper JP, Azzo W, Wang CY. 1983. Reactivity of monoclonal antibodies Leu 1 and OKT2 with malignant human lymphoid cells. Cancer 52:1369-1377.
4. Greaves MF. 1982. Phenotypic diversity of T cell leukemias. J Clin Immunol (suppl) 2:75S-80S.
5. Janossy G, Ganeshaguru K, Hoffbrand AV. 1982. Leukaemia and lymphoma: recent immunological and biochemical developments. In: Recent Advances In Haematology, Vol 3, Hoffbrand AV, ed. Edinburgh, Churchill Livingston, pp 207-231.
6. Greaves MF, Delia D, Robinson J, Sutherland R, Newman R. 1981. Exploitation of monoclonal antibodies: a "who's who" of haemopoietic malignancy. Blood Cells 7:257-280.
7. Greaves M, Delia D, Sutherland R, Rao J, Verbi W, Kemshead J, Hariri G, Goldstein G, Kung P. 1981. Expression of the OKT monoclonal antibody defined antigenic determinants in malignancy. Int J Immunopharmacol 3:283-299.
8. Greaves MF, Rao J, Hariri G, Verbi W, Catovsky D, Kung P, Goldstein G. 1981. Phenotypic heterogeneity and cellular origins of T cell malignancies. Leuk Res 5:281-299.
9. Knowles DM, Tolidjian B, Marboe CC, Mittler RS, Talle MA, Goldstein G. 1984. Distribution of antigens defined by OKB monoclonal antibodies on benign and malignant lymphoid cells and on nonlymphoid tissues. Blood 63:886-896.
10. Ritz J, Pesando JM, McConarty JN, Lazarus H, Schlossman SF.

1980. A monoclonal antibody to human acute lymphoblastic leukemia antigen. Nature 283:583-585.
11. Mertelsman R, Mertelsman I, Koziner B, Moore MAS, Clarkson BD. 1978. Improved biochemical assay for terminal deoxynucleotidyl transferase in human blood cells: results in 80 adult patients with lymphoid leukemias and malignant lymphomas in leukemic phase. Leuk Res 2:57-62.
12. Foon KA, Schroff RW, Gale RP. 1982. Surface markers on leukemia and lymphoma cells: recent advances. Blood 60:1-17.
13. Brodsky FM, Parham P, Barnstable CJ, Crumpton MJ, Bodmer WF. 1979. Hybrid myeloma monoclonal antibodies against MHC products. Immunol Rev 47:3-61.
14. Norgaard-Pedersen B, Axelsen NH, eds. 1978. Carcinoembryonic Proteins: Recent Progress, Vol 8. London, Blackwell Scientific Publications, pp 27-38.
15. Norgaard-Pedersen B, Axelsen NH, eds. 1978. Carcinoembryonic Proteins: Recent Progress, Vol 8. London, Blackwell Scientific Publications, pp 3-26.
16. Norgaard-Pedersen B, Axelsen NH, eds. 1978. Carcinoembryonic Proteins: Recent Progress, Vol 8. London, Blackwell Scientific Publications, pp 55-64.
17. Ablin RJ. 1981. Prostatic acid phosphatase: a look and word of caution. Allergol Immunopathol 9:357-358.
18. Haagensen DE Jr, Barry WF Jr, McCook CA, et al. 1980. The value of serial plasma levels of carcinoembryonic antigen and gross cyst disease fluid protein in patients with breast carcinoma and osseous metastases. Ann Surg 191:599-603.
19. Sears H, Herlyn J, DelVillano B, Steplewski Z, Koprowski H. 1982. Monoclonal antibody detection of a circulating tumor-associated antigen: II. A longitudinal evaluation of patients with colorectal cancer. J Clin Immunol 2:141-149.
20. Bast RC Jr, Klug TL, St John E, Jenison E, Niloff JM, Lazarus H, Berkowitz RS, Leavitt T, Griffiths CT, Parker L, Zurawski VR Jr, Knapp RC. 1983. A radioimmunoassay using a monoclonal antibody to monitor the course of epithelial ovarian cancer. N Engl J Med 309:883-887.
21. Goldenberg DM, Pant KD. 1976. Colonic cancer-associated antigens in a heterografted human tumor, GW-39. In: Onco-developmental gene expression, Fishman WH, Sell S, eds. New York, Academic Press, pp 617-620.
22. Hansen HJ, Snyder JJ, Miller E, Vandevoorde JP, Miller ON, Hines LR, Burns JJ. 1974. Carcinoembryonic antigen (CEA) assay. A laboratory adjunct in the diagnosis and management of cancer. Hum Pathol 5:139-147.
23. Chu TM, Holyoke ED, Murphy GP. 1974. Carcinoembryonic antigen. Current clinical status. NY State J Med 74:1388-1398.
24. Houstek J, Masopust J, Kithier K, Radlo J. 1968. Hepatocellular carcinoma in association with a specific fetal alpha-1-globulin fetoprotein. J Pediatr 72:186-193.
25. Sakuragi N. 1982. Serum SPI and hCG beta-subunit (hCG beta) levels in choriocarcinoma, invasive mole, and hydatiform mole--clinical significance of SPI/hCG beta ratio. Gynecol Oncol 13:393-398.
26. Mesa-Tejada R, personal communication.
27. Herberman RB. 1977. Immunologic tests in diagnosis of cancer. Am J Clin Pathol 68:688-698.
28. Hellstrom I, Hellstrom KE, Sjogren HO, et al. 1971. Demonstration of cell-mediated immunity to human neoplasia of various histological types. Int J Cancer 7:1-16.

29. Whittaker MG, Rees K, Clark CG. 1971. Reduced lymphocyte transformation in breast cancer. Lancet 1:892-893.
30. Miller DG. 1968. The immunologic capability of patients with lymphoma. Cancer Res 28:1441-1448.
31. Reckel RT, Harris J, Botsko E, Wellerson R, Varga S. 1985 (in press). Detection of circulating immune complexes containing Clq-IgG using a new rapid serum ELISA test system. Diag Immunol.
32. Dent PB, Louis JA, McCulloch PB, Dunnett CW, Cerottini J-C. 1980. Correlation of elevated Clq binding activity and carcinoembryonic antigen levels with clinical features and prognosis in bronchogenic carcinoma. Cancer 45:130-136.

USE OF RADIO-LABELED ANTIBODIES IN DIAGNOSIS AND STAGING OF SOLID TUMORS

SAMUEL E. HALPERN and ROBERT O. DILLMAN

Pressman and Keighley[1] demonstrated in 1948 that anti-kidney antibodies could be radio-labeled with ^{131}I without loss of immunoreactivity, and when administered to an animal, localize renal tissue. In 1953, the same investigators detected a mouse osteosarcoma using radio-labeled anti-tumor antibodies.[2] Since then, many reports have been published on uptake of radio-labeled anti-tumor antibodies in animal models.[3-5]

The use of athymic mouse models bearing human tumor xenographs extended this work to tumors of man. Using ^{125}I anti-carcinoembryonic antigen (CEA), Mach et al[6] achieved a two-fold greater tumor concentration and faster clearance of this antibody from mice than they achieved with a nonspecific globulin. Primus et al[7] showed approximately the same thing in a hamster model.

Radioimmunodetection work in humans began in the 1970s, and the first results were disappointing. Eventually, however, successful studies took place in the detection of hypernephroma[8] and with the use of antibodies against human chorionic gonadotrophin,[9] alpha-fetoprotein[10] and CEA.[11-13] It was necessary, however, to utilize electronic subtraction techniques to image most of the lesions due to the high background radioactivity. Even with subtraction, Mach et al[14] were able to detect only 11 of 27 lesions. The radiopharmaceutical concentration in the tumor averaged results, but no other lab has achieved his success rate.

In 1975, Kohler and Millstein[15] developed the hybridoma technique for producing monoclonal antibodies (MoAbs), which provided a new tool for this work. Farrands et al[16] and Mach et al[17] have successfully imaged colon tumors in humans using ^{131}I anti-CEA monoclonal antibodies. The latter investigators have also utilized ^{131}I F(ab)2 and Fab fragments.[18] Larson et al[19] have been able to image melanoma in humans using ^{131}I intact murine MoAb and ^{131}I and

^{123}I Fab preparations. While background problems decreased with use of Fab, the absolute amounts of ^{123}I in the tumors was even less than described for intact MoAb. Anti-mouse antibodies were observed in Larson and Carresquillo's studies,[20] a phenomena also observed by our group.

Work in our lab,[21] corroborated in other laboratories, indicates that dehalogenation is one of the reasons for the apparent low concentration of radio-labeled MoAbs and polyclonal antibodies in tumor tissue.[22] The free iodine leaves the tumor and is excreted in the urine. To circumvent this problem, our group (and others) have chosen to label with ^{111}In.[21-24]

The labeling with ^{111}In is not difficult; however, it does require great attention to detail. While several methods have been published, the following, which is basically a modification of that of Krejcarek and Tucker,[25] has worked well in our hands. In the initial step, DTPA is reacted with five equivolents of triethylamine, and the reaction product lyophilized and dissolved in dry acetonitrile. When this compound reacts with isobutylchoroformate, the carboxycarbonic anhydride of DTPA will be formed. The anhydride will in turn react with amine groups (principally lysine) on the antibody resulting in a side chain conjugated antibody. A large guantity of free DTPA will be formed during this reaction. The DTPA must be removed from the solution or it will compete with the conjugated protein for the ^{111}In. In the original Krejcarek and Tucker technique, this was accomplished by dialysis. It has been our observation that we cannot completely rid the reaction mixture of free DTPA by this technique. The antibody-DTPA complex is therefore separated from free DTPA by passing it through a sephadex G75 column. That antibody which elutes in the void column is pooled, and used for labeling with buffered ^{111}In. In the final step, 5mCi of carrier-free ^{111}In are reacted for 30 minutes with lmg of side chain conjugated antibody that has been mixed with equimolar amounts of human serum albumin. Subsequent purification on the sephadex G75 column cleans up the protein and the fraction eluting with the void volume is used for the studies. For best labeling efficiency, the pH should be somewhere in the vicinity of 5 or less, and under no circumtances should the pH be allowed to drop below 4.0. Should this happen, the immunoreactivity of the molecule will continue to be approximately that prior to the insult; however, the protein will be denatured and the in vivo kinetics altered. A high liver uptake of ^{111}In is generally the result of such damage. It should be remembered that extremely pure ^{111}In should be utilized in preparation of the radiopharmaceutical, ie, free of competing ions, and that no more than one side chain should be put on one MoAb molecule.

If the preparation is made correctly, the kinetics shown in Figure 1a and 1b will prevail. In this particular study, the ^{111}In preparation was administered to nude mice implanted with a CEA-producing human colon tumor. These animals were followed for seven days. The same MoAb was endogeneously labeled with ^{75}Se and thus represented a MoAb which had not gone through the labeling process. The ^{75}Se-labeled moiety was administered to parallel groups of animals also bearing this specific colon tumor. The results shown in Figure 1 are nearly identical, the major differences occurring in the liver where there was an increased concentration of ^{111}In compared to the ^{75}Se moiety, and in the tumor where there was a greater concentration of the endogenously labeled antibody. Part of the reason for the higher concentration of ^{75}Se into the tumor was due to the fact that the animals receiving this radiopharmaceutical had smaller tumors, therefore a better blood supply, and concentrated the radiopharmaceutical to a greater degree based upon this variable. However, it should be pointed out that there was some difficulty in the ^{111}In labeling process, and this also led to the higher concentrations in the liver and to some degree the lower concentrations of ^{111}In in the tumor. Subsequent to this, we have reduced the number of side chains on the antibody, and now have a preparation which gives virtually identical results with the ^{75}Se-labeled moiety.

The stability of the ^{111}In label was assessed by several different mechanisms. In the most sophisticated of these an animal was administered 50uCi of ^{111}In MoAb 24 hours prior to its exsanguination. The blood of this animal was then administered to both normal and tumor-bearing mice. These were sacrificed at 4 and 24 hours. The distribution was the same in the recipients as it was in the donor animals.

Finally, it was proven in a tumor model experiment that a ^{111}In-labeled MoAb specific for the tumor concentrated in that a.

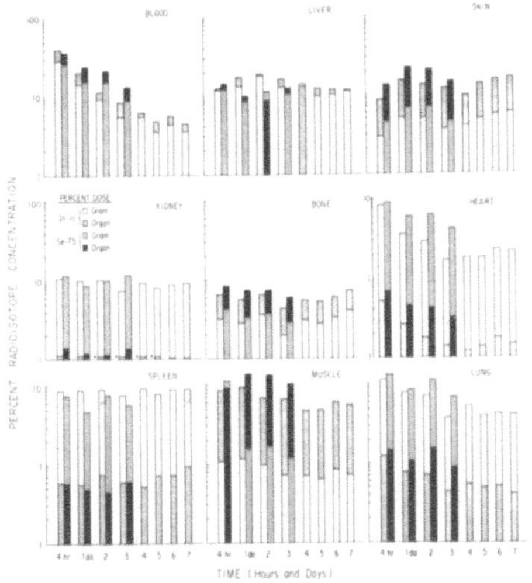

b.

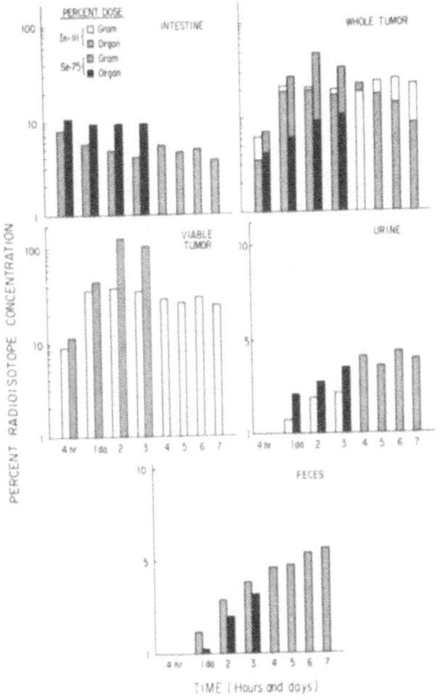

FIGURE 1. Distribution of ^{111}In versus ^{75}Se-labelled MoAbs in nude mouse model. Note similarity of distribution of the two radiopharmaceuticals.

tumor to a higher degree than a nonspecific MoAb (also labeled with ^{111}In).

HUMAN SCANNING

Radioimmunoimaging of humans in our laboratory has involved mostly patients having metastatic malignant melanoma. Both the P-96.5 MoAb, which targets a 97,000 molecular weight cell surface antigen and a MoAb against the so-called high molecular weight antigen have been ^{111}In-labeled and used as radiopharmaceuticals. In a majority of cases we have used 5mCi of ^{111}In, and the quantity of protein associated with it has varied from 1mg to 20mg.

Our results with the 96.5 MoAb have been encouraging to date. We have shown that the kinetics and distribution of the radiopharmaceutical can be altered by varying the absolute mass of antibody injected. The disappearance of the ^{111}In from the vascular compartment is much faster when low MoAb mass is administered than following high MoAb dose. The administration of 1mg or less of the antibody results in rapid and marked liver, spleen and bone marrow uptake of the radiopharmaceutical. There also seems to be a much better chance of detecting the tumor when a larger MoAb mass is administered. Overall, we have imaged approximately 60% of the known lesions with this MoAb. In those patients that received between 10mg and 20mg of the protein, 80% or greater of the lesions were seen. Our patients were not selected for presence of antigen on the tumor.

Figure 2 is typical of the scans using ^{111}In-P-96.5 MoAb. Note the high concentrations in the liver and spleen. It is estimated that approximately 15% of the radiopharmaceutical is in the liver. Occasionally there is also a problem from radiopharmaceutical in the gastrointestinal tract. Since the majority of this is in the small intestine, it is sometimes necessary to image on successive days to determine if a radioactive site is a lesion or simply bowel activity. SPECT imaging appears helpful in delineating lesions that are vague on planar images. Subtraction techniques have not been used with ^{111}In imaging; however, it would be possible to use them if it became desirable.

One of the advantages of the melanoma system is the virtual absence of circulating antigen. This is important since studies in our laboratory indicate that, at least in the nude mouse model,

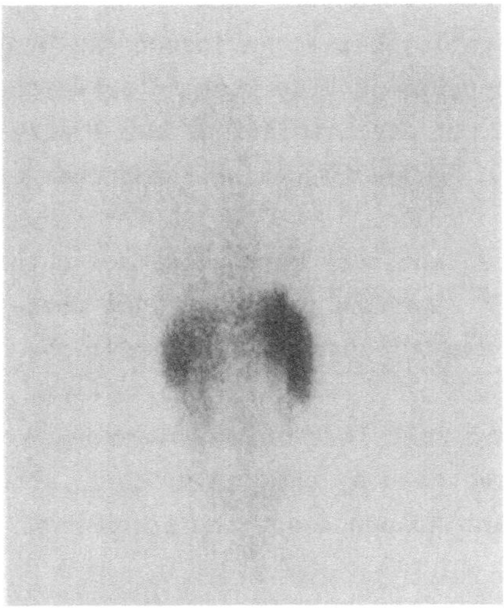

FIGURE 2. Distribution of ^{111}In-P-96.5 anti-melanoma MoAb. The uptake in the liver and spleen are normal findings with this particular antibody.

circulating antigen results in the formation of immune complexes which are quickly removed by the liver. The end result is a very high liver concentration of radioactivity with a reduction in tracer concentration by the tumor. Circulating antigen is not considered to pose an imaging problem by investigators who use ^{131}I-MoAb. It is the opinion of the authors, however, based upon data developed in the nude mouse model, that the reason high liver activity is not observed in these patients is that the immune complexes are rapidly dehalogenated with excretion of the iodine in the urine. Thus, the liver appears not to have concentrated the labeled MoAb. In short, the effect of complex formation is only observed when the label is stable.

Radioimmunoimaging employing ^{111}In as the radionuclide has much to recommend it in comparison with ^{131}I. It produces nearly two photons per disintegration with energy levels of 173 and 247 KeV. Both of these photons are detectable with a standard gamma camera and allow medium energy collimation. The type of collimation used is very important as regards resolution of the lesion. Imaging ^{131}I necessitates use of a high energy collimator. This degrades the image.

The photon flux produced by ^{111}In is such that SPECT imaging, which is highly dependent upon statistical significance of counts, becomes very easy. The exact opposite is true with ^{131}I, which not only has fewer photons available per disintegration, but a very low scintillation crystal efficiency, further reducing the number of detectable photons.

^{111}In can be chelated onto an antibody without damaging the protein when care is taken in the labeling process. Once there, it is tightly bound and is not removed by enzymatic action in the manner of halides.

Finally, the 2.8 day physical half life of ^{111}In matches well with the incorporation rate of the MoAb by the tumor. The latter is true, of course, only of intact MoAb and not the fragments.

OTHER LABELED ANTIBODIES

Studies with ZME-018

ZME-018 is an IgG2A MoAb which targets the so-called high molecular weight antigen on the surface of the melanoma cell. Human studies to date have indicated that it has a different in vivo distribution than P-96.5. The spleen becomes quite radioactive very early following administration of ^{111}In-AME-018. The liver, however, appears to be less radioactive than with P-96.5. To date we have had good results in imaging with this MoAb, but it is too early to make any statement as to how well it will work.

Other antibodies

Figure 3 shows an image of an anti-prostatic acid phosphatase MoAb labeled with ^{111}In (5mg 2.5mCi) in a patient with prostatic carcinoma. Two bony lesions are obvious. What is not obvious is that multiple bony metastases exist in this patient which were not imaged. Once again, the pattern of distribution of this radiopharmaceutical is different from that of the other two described. There is a considerable degree of bone marrow uptake, yet unlike ZME-018, the spleen is only moderately radioactive. Thus far, the prostatic acid phosphatase antibody has not proven as efficacious as the melanoma antibodies; however, dose escalation ala P-96.5 has not yet been performed.

Monoclonal anti-tumor antibodies that target white cells

Our first efforts in radioimmunoimaging began with a ^{111}In anti-CEA antibody.[26] Following administration of the radio-

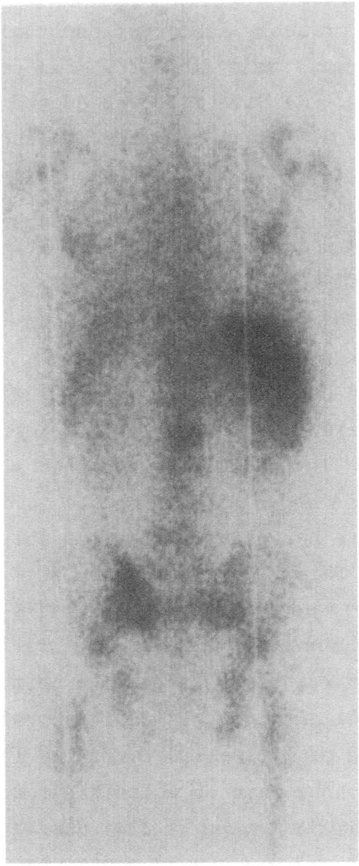

FIGURE 3. Distribution of ^{111}In anti-prostatic acid phosphatase antibody in a patient with metastic prostate carcinoma. Note uptake in the sacrum. The patient had other metastases which were not visualized with the antibody.

pharmaceutical, the patient developed chills and fever necessitating cessation of infusion. Scanning was performed immediately following recuperation of the patient (about one half hour later). Marked uptake of the ^{111}In was observed in the reticuloendothelial organs. None of the colon tumor metastases in the liver concentrated the radiopharmaceutical. In fact, the scans showed diminished uptake of ^{111}In in the metastases while the areas of increased uptake represented the normal tissue. It was later discovered that this MoAb targeted white blood cells in the vascular compartment. These cells were removed by the reticuloendothelial system as evidenced by a rapid drop in the white cell count in these patients. The leukocytes were probably destroyed and their contents liberated into the circulation. This, in turn, induced a pyrogen-type reaction in the patients. We have since abandoned use of this MoAb, but the message was clear. If solid tumor imaging is the goal, MoAbs must be carefully screened to exclude reactivity with circulating cells.

Figure 4 is an example of a scan using ^{111}In-labeled T-101 MoAb[27] in patients with T-cell lymphoma.

One mg of ^{111}In-T-101 was infused followed by 500mg of unlabeled T-101 MoAb over the next 24 hours. This patient was scanned immediately and over a period of days following the radiopharmaceutical. Note the marked uptake in the lymph nodes. Large concentrations of ^{111}In also occurred in the spleen and other reticuloendothelial organs. The lymph nodes did not become obvious until 24 hours post-infusion, and were not at their maximum intensity until 48 hours post-injection. This finding suggests that the antibody may not have arrived in these nodes as a single entity, but rather conjoined to the T cell which bore the specific antigen. This same patient was treated again three weeks later. At this time the 500mg dose of unlabeled T-101 antibody was administered over a 23 hour period followed by 1mg of ^{111}In-T-101 over the last hour. This protocol markedly reduced the rate at which the radiopharmaceutical left the vascular compartment and further decreased the radiopharmaceutical uptake in the spleen. By 72 hours the

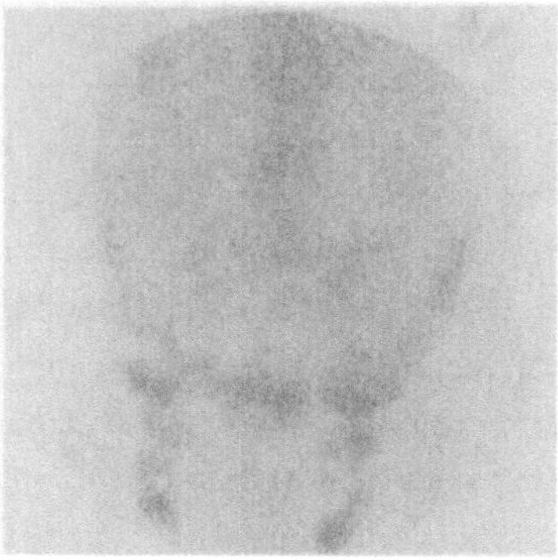

FIGURE 4. Note marked uptake of ^{111}In-T-101 antibody in inguinal lymph nodes in a patient with cutaneous T cell lymphoma. Most of the nodes were quite small (0.5 cm diameter).

lymph nodes previously seen were again apparent and to approximately the same intensity seen in the first administration.

The next patient had the ^{111}In-T-101 MoAb administered following a 500mg dose of cold T-101. There was no evidence of nodal activity in this patient, probably because his disease was not far advanced. The usual deposits of the ^{111}In were observed, however. Three weeks later, the patient received the ^{111}In-T-101 antibody over a period of one hour followed by a 500mg dose infused over the next 23 hours. The scan indicated a very rapid clearing of the radiopharmaceutical with deposit of large amounts of the radiopharmaceutical in the liver. The blood disappearance curves indicated a very rapid disappearance of the ^{111}In from the vascular compartment. These findings were indicative of immune complex formation and clearance of the complexes by the liver. Approximately one week later, the patient developed signs and symptoms of immune complex disease. He responded to aspirin and has done well since. Serological tests confirmed he had high levels of anti-mouse antibodies at the time of the second infusion.

In summary, we have developed a technique for applying ^{111}In to monoclonal anti-tumor antibodies and have successfully targeted tumor in melanoma, prostate carcinoma, and T-cell lymphoma. The technique looks promising at this time as a means of detection of tumor, however, a great deal more work needs to be performed prior to radioimmunoimaging becomes a routine clinical procedure.

REFERENCES

1. Pressman D, Keighley G. 1948. The zone of activity of antibodies as destermined by the use of radioactive tracers; the zone of activity of nephrotoxic antikidney serum. J Immunol 59:141-146.
2. Pressman D, Korngold L. 1953. The in vivo localization of anti-Wagner osteogenic sarcoma antibodies. Cancer 6:619-623.
3. Korngold L, Pressman D. 1954. The localization of anti-lymphosarcoma antibodies in the Murphy lymphosarcoma of the rat. Cancer Res 14:96-99.
4. Day ED, Planisek JA, Pressman D. 1960. Localization of radioiodinated antibodies in rats bearing tumors induced by N-2-Fluorenylacetamide. J Natl Cancer Inst 25:787-802.
5. Kyogoku M, Yagi Y, Planinsek J, Pressman D. 1964. Localizing properties of anti-rat hepatoma antibodies in vivo. Cancer Res 24:268-279.
6. Mach JP, Carrel S, Merenda C, et al. 1974. In vivo localization of radiolabeled antibodies to carcinoembryonic antigen in human colon carcinoma grafted into nude mice. Nature 248:704-706.

7. Primus FJ, MacDonald R, Goldenberg DM, Hansen HJ. 1977. Localization of the W-39 tumors in hamsters by affinity-purified antibody to carcinoembryonic antigen. Cancer Res 37:1544-1547.
8. Belitsky P, Ghose T, Aguino J, et al. 1978. Radionuclide imaging of metastases from renal cell carcinoma by ^{131}I-labeled anti-tumor antibody. Radiology 126:515-517.
9. Jaradpour N, Kim EE, DeLand FH, Salyer JP, Shah U, Goldenberg DM. 1981. The role of radioimmunodetection in the management of testicular cancer. J Am Med Assoc 246:45-49.
10. Koji T, Ishii T, Munehisa Y, et al. 1980. Localization of radioiodinated antibody to alpha feto protein. Antibody treatment of a hepatoma patient. Cancer Res 40:3013-3015.
11. Goldenberg DM, DeLand F, Kim E, et al. 1978. Use of radiolabeled antibodies to carcinoembryonic antigen for the detection and localization of diverse cancers by external photoscanning. N Engl J Med 298:1384-1388.
12. Kim EE, DeLand FH, Casper S, et al. 1980. Radioimmunodetection of colorectal cancer. Cancer 45:1243-1247.
13. Van Nagell JR, Kim E, Casper S, et al. 1980. Radioimmunodetection of primary and metastatic ovarian cancer using radiolabeled antibodies to carcinoembryonic antigen. Cancer Res 40:502-506.
14. Mach JP, Carrel S, Forni M, et al. 1980. Tumor localization of radiolabeled antibodies against carcinoembryonic antigen in patients with carcinoma. N Engl J Med 303:5-10.
15. Kohler G, Milstein C. 1975. Continuous cultures of fused cells secreting antibody of predetermined specificity. Nature 256:495-497.
16. Farrands PA, Pimm MV, Embleton MJ, et al. 1982. Radioimmunodetection of human colorectal cancers by an antitumour monoclonal antibody. Lancet 2:8295-8298.
17. Mach JP, Buchegger F, Forni M, et al. 1981. Use of radiolabelled monoclonal anti-CEA antibodies for the detection of human carcinomas by external photoscanning and tomoscintigraphy. Immunol Today 2:239-249, 1981.
18. Delaloye B, Bischof-Delaloye A, Grob JPh, Buchegger F, Halpern S, Fliedner VV, Mach JP. 1984. SPECT with I-123 labeled F(ab)2 fragments from monoclonal antibodies in colon carcinoma. J Nucl Med 25:1-17.
19. Larson SM, Brown JP, Wright PW, Carrasquillo JA, Hellstrom I, Hellstrom KE. 1983. Imaging of melanoma with I-131-labeled monoclonal antibodies. J Nucl Med 24:123-129.
20. Larson SM. Personal Communication.
21. Halpern S, Stern P, Hagan P, et al. 1983. The labeling of monoclonal antibodies with ^{111}Indium: technique and advantages compared to radioiodine labeling. In: Burchiel and Rhodes (ed). Elsevier Press, pp 197-205.
22. Sullivan DC, Silva JS, Cox CE, et al. 1982. Localization of I-131 labeled goat and primate anti carcinoembryonic antigen (CEA) antibodies in patients with cancer. Invest Radiol 17:350-355.
23. Halpern SE, Hagan PL., Garver PR, et al. 1983. Stability, characterization and kinetics of ^{111}In-labeled monoclonal antibodies in normal animals and nude mouse-human tumor models. Cancer Res 43:5347-5355.
24. Halpern SE, Dillman RO, Hagan PL. 1983. The problems and promise of monoclonal antitumor antibodies. Diag Imag 5:47-49.
25. Krejcarek GE, Tucker KL. 1977. Covalent attachment of chelating groups to macromolecules. Biochem Biophys Res Com 77:581-

585.
26. Dillman RO, Beauregard JC, Sobol RE, Royston I, Bartholomew RM, Hagan PL, Halpern SE. 1984. Lack of radioimmunodetection and complications associated with monoclonal anticarcinoembryonic antigen antibody cross-reactivity with an antigen on circulating cells. Cancer Res 44:2214-2218.
27. Dillman RO, Shawler DL, Dillman JB, Royston I. 1984. Therapy of chronic leukemia and cutaneous T-cell lymphoma with T-101 monoclonal antibody. J Clin Oncol 2:881-891.

FLOW CYTOMETRY IN LYMPHOMA/LEUKEMIA DIAGNOSIS

JOHN W. PARKER

INTRODUCTION

As Robert Lukes' first fellow at USC, in 1964, and his associate since then, it is a great pleasure to see him honored by this symposium. Much of what is being presented here has been influenced directly or indirectly by his ideas and concepts of the biology of lymphomas. His hypothesis of blocks in transformation as a mechanism for the development of follicular center cell lymphomas (Lukes and Collins) is now widely accepted. Parallel findings by other investigators make it now common to speak of impairment in differentiation ("frozen stages") to explain the derivation of cells in hematopoietic neoplasms.[1,2] All of the answers are not in, but no matter what the final outcome, Dr. Lukes' ideas and proposals have stimulated many investigators, pathologists and clinicians to change their thinking about lymphomas.

A very practical offshoot of the concept that lymphomas and leukemias represent blocks in differentiation has been the development of increasingly sophisticated methods for phenotyping lymphoma/leukemia cells. This phenotyping has proven of clinical value in several conditions, particularly acute lymphocytic leukemia of childhood.

When we first began to apply the then available markers to phenotyping lymphomas, approximately ten years ago, we relied on rosetting techniques, immunofluorescence and cytochemistry. These proved useful[3] but were limited in their specificity for lymphocyte subsets. In 1979 when Koehler and Millstein[4] published their hybridoma methodology for producing monoclonal antibodies, the field was ripe for their application to lymphoma/leukemia cell phenotyping. In large degree this was because a new generation of cytofluorographs were being developed by instrument manufacturers for use in clinical laboratories. These new clinical cytofluorographs are less expensive, easier to use, have easier maintenance and less down time than the more sophisticated cell sorters in use for several years in research laboratories. The marriage of these new reagents and new instruments has provided a practical approach to phenotyping lymphocytes in lymphoma/leukemia and in cetain infectious diseases, particularly AIDS. However, we have only seen the beginning. The offspring from this marriage will certainly be many since essentially any fluorescent probe can be used to characterize a dispersed suspension of particles whether they be cells, sub-cellular particles or organisms. Thus we are at the threshold of another explosion in the application of new technology to clinical laboratory medicine.

Because our group at USC had several years experience with phenotyping lymphoma and leukemia cells prior to monoclonal antibodies, it was natural for us to use these new reagents and flow cytometry. Since 1981 when we acquired an Ortho Spectrum 3 Cytofluorograph, my laboratory has phenotyped over 6000 specimens including blood, lymphoid tissue, bone marrow, non-lymphoid tissues, body fluids (effusions, CSF, bronchial lavages, etc.). The phenotyping results reported by my USC colleagues in this symposium were all performed in my laboratory.

Why Phenotype? The classifications and nomenclatures for the lymphoproliferative disorders have been cumbersome and difficult to utilize because of their heterogeneity and, until recently, the application of morphological criteria alone. Early immunophenotyping of acute lymphocytic leukemia (ALL) indicated clinical usefulness in diagnosis, prognosis and choice of therapy. If we accept the concept that lymphomas represent arrests in lymphocyte transformation or differentiation, then it follows that precise staging of the arrest by correlating the lymphoma phenotype with a stage of lymphocyte differentiation will be of potential value, even if only in aiding understanding. The use of monoclonal antibodies in conjunction with flow cytometry allows us to phenotype with more precision.

MONOCLONAL ANTIBODIES

Many monoclonal antibodies have been produced since hybridoma technology became available, and the number of commercially available monoclonal antibodies is increasing at a rapid rate. Some are discussed in recent reviews.[5,6] These antibodies can be used to phenotype lymphocytes in a variety of diseases. Unfortunately there has been a tendency to equate phenotype with function, and although there are demonstrated associations, we are only at the beginning of our understanding of the phenotypic and functional heterogeneity of lymphoid and myeloid cells and histiocytes. Because of the increasing number of probes, the complexity of this information will increase.

It has already been demonstrated that immunological phenotyping has therapeutic value in acute lymphocytic leukemia, and our sophistication in utilizing these antibodies is increasing at a logarithmic rate.

Cell Type Specificity of Monoclonal Antibodies. Initial work by Reinherz et al, suggested that monoclonal antibodies raised against T-cell differentiation antigens had significant specificity for certain subsets of lymphocytes with functional homogeneity, ie, OKT 4-positive "helper" cells, OKT 8-positive "suppressor" cells.[7] From this and other studies have come a variety of T-cell differentiation maps. However, it has become clear with more extensive clinical application of these antibodies that cell type specificity is not precise. For example, initial impressions that OKT 9 and OKT 10 antibodies were specific for prothymocytes or progenitor cells in the T-cell system have proven to be in error. OKT 9 recognizes a transferin receptor and is present on a variety of activated lymphocytes and other cells. OKT 10 appears to recognize activated or proliferating T and B lymphocytes and other cells.

In the original testing of antibodies by investigators, an antibody may identify a limited range of normal cell types. A more extensive study of a variety of normal and diseased tissues by multiple investigators demonstrates that certain antigen epitopes are present on a larger range of cell types than originally suspected. This should not be discouraging and actually can be used to advantage. It is already clear that single antibodies for phenotyping are insufficient, and panels of antibodies will produce extended phenotypes which are useful diagnostically, particularly in neoplasms. It should not surprise us that tumor cells express a range of antigens, most of them differentiation antigens, since it is increasingly clear that undifferentiated cells may upon occasion express late differentiation antigens because of inappropriate gene activation.

The exquisite degree of epitope specificity of these reagents may also present a problem in interpretation since antibodies thought equivalent may actually recognize different epitopes on the same antigen. This may lead to confusion in clinical situations since results will depend on the reagents used. Certain diseases may reflect one epitope of a cellular antigen, but not the others.[8]

Until there is more clinical experience with the antibodies being used, cell specificity claims should be viewed with open-minded skepticism, remembering that while the antibodies have a high degree of antigen specificity, the restriction of antigens to cell types is not necessarily highly specific.

FLOW CYTOMETRY

Flow cytometers are used in most hematology laboratories for cell counting and sizing. A new generation of flow cytometers has now entered the clinical laboratory.[9] These measure fluorescence intensity as well as light scatter. By counting thousands of cells per second and utilizing fluorescent probes, these instruments are able to detect and quantitate an increasing range of cell populations. Any cell suspension whether it comes directly as a suspension from body fluids or is man-made from dispersed tissues, can be analyzed by these flow cytometers. The spectrum of fluorescent probes is almost unlimited, requiring only that a reagent (whether an antibody, antigen, or some other specific probe) be conjugated to a fluorochrome or be a fluorochrome. The original flow cytometers provided by Wallace Coulter 25 years ago have been improved by advances in electronics and computers so that the cytofluorographs presently available are quite sophisticated. These instruments are powered by a light source which is either a laser or mercury arc lamp and have electronics which convert light scatter and fluorescence impuses to digital signals. The latter are collected and analyzed by computer systems which also control the instrument operation.

Light Scatter. As the cell enters the focused light beam, light is scattered in an arc of 360°. Current commercial instruments measure light scatter signals generated by photodetectors placed in front of the beam (forward or low angle scatter) and at 90° to the light beam (right angle scatter). The forward angle scatter is 2°-10° and gives information regarding the cell size.

Right angle scatter provides information about the external and internal cellular structure and granularity, particularly the nuclear shape. By combining forward angle and right angle light scatter measurements, a cytogram is provided which allows identification of different cell populations. Of much use in this regard is the cytogram presented by peripheral blood leukocytes in which lymphocytes, monocytes, and granulocytes can be identified by their light scatter characteristics.[10]

The current generation of instruments allows one to gate a specific population in the cytogram for analysis. The populations are outlined by a cursor, and only those cells targeted are analyzed. Dead cells are also identifiable and can be excluded electronically.

Fluorescence. Photo detectors are placed at a 90° angle to incident light, providing a great degree of sensitivity in measuring fluorescence. It has been estimated that the human eye requires 2300 to 2500 molecules of fluorochrome to identify it as positive; whereas the flow cytometer can detect between 800 and 2000 fluorochrome molecules. This may be of particular value when cell surface antigens are present in smaller than normal quantities, eg, in chronic lymphocytic leukemia (CLL), and might falsely be labelled as null cells by visual methods.[11] However, in spite of the sensitivity of this approach there are disadvantages, since the instrument detects only fluorescence and cannot record the distribution of fluorescent molecules on each cell surface or determine whether the fluorescence is on the surface or inside the cell. The technologist viewing immunofluorescence specimens through a microscope is able to make some judgements as to whether cells are alive or dead, whether the correct cell population is being analyzed and whether a fluorescent cell looks "real" or is nonspecifically labelled. This is balanced by the speed of gathering large amounts of quantitative data with a cytometer and the light scatter characteristics of different viable cells and dead cells.

Multiple color analysis is possible by using fluorochromes stimulated at the same wavelength but emitting at different wavelengths or by using more than one laser with different exciting lines. It can be assumed that technology will ultimately develop so that a large number of different fluorochromes can be analyzed at the same time by using both of the principles above. The advantages of this approach are that each cell poulation under study can be subdivided into multiple phenotypes based on positive and negative results with each fluorochrome labelled probe. An example already in use is the selective analysis of subpopulations of lymphocytes from patients with leukemias and lymphomas. The neoplastic population may be selected with a specific antibody and then analyzed for DNA content.

Fluorescent signals strike photodetectors and are amplified, analyzed and viewed on display screens. A fluorescence histogram from an antibody analysis of a cell suspension shows not only the percentage of positive and negative cells but also a display of the fluorescence intensity for the positive cells. This may be an advantage in distinguishing between different types of leukemia because of differences in the shape of fluorescence histograms.

Of particular value in the development of computers associated with these instruments is the ability of some to store data "list mode." In other words, all of the signals are stored so that in retrospect a population can be redisplayed and selective information, the importance of which was not recognized in the initial analysis, can be reanalyzed.

Overall this new technology for analysis of cells using a range of probes of varying specificity has almost unlimited potential. The potential impact on clinical laboratory medicine is immense because fluorescent probes for cell components, DNA, chromosomes, genes, oncogenes, etc., can be used with flow cytometry.

The features of flow cytometry that have particular relevance in terms of the advantages of flow cytometry in characterizing lymphocytes, particularly neoplastic ones include: (1) the simplicity and rapidity of fluorescence labelling methods; (2) collection of quantitative data on single cells; (3) detection of small numbers of abnormal cells in body fluids; (4) accumulation and correlation of several parameters on the same specimen; (5) antibody panel phenotyping of cell populations; (6) necessity for only small numbers of cells in aliquots analyzed; (7) rapid analysis; (10,000 cells/sec) and (8) greater statistical significance since many more cells can be analyzed than with manual/visual methods.[11]

LYMPHOMAS AND LEUKEMIAS

Acute Lymphocytic Leukemia (ALL). Nowhere has it been more apparent than in ALL that immunological phenotyping of leukemia cells has clinical relevance.

Although ALL was previously considered a uniformly fatal disease, phenotyping results have made it clear that at least five or six different lymphocyte cell types are involved[12,13] and that prognosis and choice of therapy are related to the phenotype.[14-16] The hoped-for ultimate outcome, of course, is that panels of markers (immunological, biochemical and morphological) will eventually be identified for all types of lymphoma/leukemia, and that effective, specific therapy will be tailored for each phenotype.

Subclassification within the T-ALL type has been reported using monoclonal antibodies directed against different T-cell antigens.[7] E rosette-forming cells from several patients with T-ALL, exposed to a panel of antibodies which identify T cell "differentiation antigens," were found to have different phenotypes which corresponded to stages in thymocyte differentiation. Therefore it appears that, even within the supposedly homogeneous T-ALL cells, there is phenotypic heterogeneity.

These studies of ALL cells indicate that the antigens present seem to be normal differentiation antigens rather than "tumor-specific" antigens. The common ALL antigen (cALLa), originally thought specific for ALL cells, is now known to be present on primitive cells in fetal and regenerating bone marrow, some normal blood lymphocytes and cells in reactive lymphoid tissue. It is probably an early B lymphocyte differentiation antigen, although it is also present on endothelial cells in lymph nodes. The antigens found on T-ALL cells are also apparently normal differentiation antigens.

These findings are consistent with results of tumor immunology studies in general, ie, so-called tumor-specific antigens appear to be only "tumor associated" and represent the expression of oncofetal antigens not usually expressed on differentiated cells. Nevertheless, even though tumor-specific neo-antigens may not exist, the potential value of monoclonal antibodies in identifying subtypes of leukemias and lymphomas within major classes is great. They may be particularly valuable in identifying the cell lineage of poorly differentiated cells. Lineage switches in acute leukemia are being well documented and emphasize the necessity for individualizing therapy.[17]

Lineage Switch in Acute Leukemia. Although not common, cases have been reported in which patients with childhood leukemia in marrow relapse have undergone a lineage switch (lymphoid to myeloid or the reverse). The switch from acute lymphoblastic leukemia, the primary diagnosis, to acute nonlymphoblastic leukemia appears to occur more often than the reverse. This is obviously important for effective therapy since, although the children respond to lineage specific multi-agent chemotherapy at the time of initial diagnosis and achieve complete remission, they require specific treatment for the new phenotype in order to achieve second remission. Of the patients reported undergoing lineage switches, most appear to have initial T cell phenotypes originally and convert to myeloblastic proliferations, suggesting that the T lymphoblasts may have the potential for myeloid differentiation or that there may be a multipotential progenitor cell capable of both T lymphoblast and myeloblast differentiation.[17,18]

Heterogeneity of stem cells is seen in patients with acute nonlymphocytic leukemia.[19] This heterogeneity might be expanded if neoplastic transformation effects a progenitor cell capable of differentiating into either myeloid or lymphoid cells. Generally there is lineage fidelity in leukemic patients, but there are several reports of simultaneous or sequential expression of lymphoid to myeloid phenotypic markers in leukemia and fairly numerous reports of lymphoblastic crisis in chronic myelogeneous leukemia.[20,21] The absence of karyotypic changes in certain patients who undergo lineage switches might suggest that a single clone is capable of either lymphoid or myeloid differentiation. This is supported by the observation that chronic myeloid leukemia has the potential for expressing both lymphoid and myeloid phenotypes in blast crisis.

These observations emphasize the need for phenotypic characterization of leukemic cells if therapy is to be tailored to the cell type involved.

Non-Hodgkin's Lymphomas and Lymphocytic Leukemias. Less is known about the clinical value of phenotyping lymphoma cells with monoclonal antibodies, but the importance of surface marker analysis in determining prognosis in B cell lymphomas is apparent.[22,23]

The value of phenotyping B cell lymphomas relates to our ability to establish their clonal character by detecting a predominant cytoplasmic or surface heavy and/or light chain.[24] Unfortunately, it is generally not possible to establish clonality with the same degree of certainty in T cell proliferations. Nevertheless, early studies of certain types of T cell lymphoma and leukemia have suggested that there are restricted immunological phenotypes.[25,26] Most T-ALL's phenotype as early pre-T cells or prothymocytes, T-CLL's as helper/inducer (T4) or suppressor/cytotoxic (T8) T cells; cutaneous lymphomas as helper cells; convoluted T cell leukemia/lymphomas as early thymocytes or prothymocytes; and T immunoblastic sarcomas as common or mature thymocytes or T lymphocytes.[25] Some of these neoplastic cells also show in vitro functional activity which is consistent with the phenotype, eg, the helper activity of Sezary cells. However, there is considerable immunophenotypic heterogeneity in this group of diseases, not readily apparent from morphology and histochemistry.[27] Current morphological criteria may not be sufficient to detect immunophenotypic differences which have clinical importance, but review of phenotypically defined groups may help to refine morphologic criteria amd make them more predictive. This approach will require the study of large numbers of patients over a period of several years to determine the clinical significance of phenotyping.

The current availability of monoclonal antibodies directed against both T and B cell differentiation antigens has increased the potential for immunophenotyping, but at the same time has infinitely expanded the potential number of subtypes of lymphoma within a single cytological type. Ideally the goal is to identify patients with lymphomas who will respond well to conventional therapy from those who will do poorly and therefore require more aggressive therapy.

Clonal Excess. In addition to the capacity of flow cytometers to characterize lymphoma and leukemia cells that may be present in significant numbers in the peripheral blood, lymphoid tissue and body fluids, the sensitivity of flow cytometry with highly specific antibodies allows one to detect quite small numbers of abnormal cells intermixed with normal cells (one labelled cell in 10^5 cells).[28] This of course depends on the availability of an antibody that recognizes a specific tumor-associated antigen. The most convincing example of this sensitivity is the detection of small numbers of neoplastic B lymphocytes in the peripheral blood in patients with B cell leukemia/lymphoma because of the "monoclonality" of their surface membrane immunoglobulin (SIg). The presence of monoclonal B cells with only one type of surface membrane light chain (kappa or lambda) in peripheral blood upsets the normal ratio of kappa to lambda SIg-bearing B cells. By most techniques there must be a sufficient number of these monoclonal B cells in blood to cause a detectable change in the ratio. Using flow cytometry, which allows the quantitation of not only the number of fluorescing cells, but the amount of surface immunoglobulin, one can demonstrate an excess of lymphocytes bearing one light chain or the other (clonal excess) even in the presence of a predominant population of normal B lymphocytes.[28] The sensitivity of this method makes it possible to detect small numbers of B cells with monoclonal surface Ig in patients who have lymphomas but do not have morphologically detectable circulating lymphoma cells and to detect the early reappearance of neoplastic B cells in relapsing leukemia or lymphoma patients.

Phenotyping Results (USC). For the past three years we have phenotyped lymphoid cell suspensions and peripheral blood lymphocytes from patients with lymphoma and leukemia, using monoclonal antibodies and cytofluorographic analysis. A panel of the antibodies which includes OKT 3, 4, 6, 8, 10, OKIa, OKMI (Ortho Diagnostics), J-5 (cALLa) (Coulter), anti-Ig, anti-kappa, anti-lambda heteroantisera (Tago), and selectively Bl, B2, My4, My7, Mol, Mo2 (Coulter), B7 (Ortho) has been used for cytofluorographic analysis of a large number of specimens from this group of patients. The phenotypes generated are being correlated with clinical features, response to therapy, and survival as an ongoing long-term study.

As with any new technology utilizing new reagents, it is essential that reagents and methods be standardized and normal ranges established. Although there are a few reports of normal values for peripheral blood, these are generally not based on large numbers of subjects or very many antibodies.[29] There is some evidence that there may be gender differences in the expression of certain T cell antigens and that there may be decreases in certain subsets with age.[29] It will take time to accumulate data on healthy donors of all ages, sexes and ethnic groups for each of the many antibodies available for use in disease studies. Additionally, antibodies from different laboratories and commercial suppliers said to have the same or similar cell specificities must be compared for evaluation of results from different institutions.

We have phenotyped a group of healthy donors with a panel of antibodies and have established normal ranges (Table 1). Since the results tend not to show Gaussian distribution curves (also noted by others,[29,30]) it was necessary to use non-parametric statistical methods to establish normal ranges. In general, differences between males and females have not been statistically significant.

We have found that in the case of B cell phenotyping, flow cytometry and visual immunofluorescence results generally agree, and E rosette scores are also in general agreement with both OKT 3 and 11 scores, although OKT 11 is reported to be specific for the sheep erythrocyte receptor.

A perennial problem in studying cell suspensions is the mixing that occurs when the suspensions are prepared. In the case of lymph nodes, large and small lymphocytes, large and small lymphoma/

Table 1. Lymphocyte Subclasses Showing Normal Ranges in Adults 20-50 Years of Age--Percent and Absolute Numbers of Labelled Cells

	Females (n=73)		Males (n=40)	
Antibody	Percent	Absolute Numbers/mm^3	Percent	Absolute Numbers/mm^3
OKT 3	60-81	959-2509	52-84	822-2641
T 11	69-91	958-2484	62-90	910-3495
T 4	32-56	489-1518	31-53	528-1804
T 8	16-37	304-909	19-45	327-1223
T 4/8	0.9-3.3	0.9-3.3	0.8-2.6	0.83-2.6
T 6	0-5	0-91	0-6	0-106
T 10	0-21	0-452	3-33	50-1103
SIg (PV)	7-31	140-678	6-40	125-932
			4-19	
SIg (kappa)	4-19	88-410	3-19	84-475
	2-14			
SIg (lambda)	0-15	45-343	2-17	48-393
Ia	0-6	0-294	0-20	30-451
cALLa	0-16	0-188	0-16	0-562
OKM_1		0-334		0-274
WBC		3930-9635		4115-10355
Lymphocytes		1326-3214		1360-3727

leukemia cells, granulocytes, monocytes, macrophages, stromal cells etc. may all be present in the suspension. Removal of the unwanted cells by various separation techniques may also remove the cells of interest, or their presence may cloud the results of antibody analysis. Fortunately light scatter analysis allows the separation of lymphocytes, granulocytes, monocytes and erythrocytes. Another problem caused by cell suspension heterogeneity is the general inability to distinguish lymphoma/leukemia cells from residual or normal or reactive lymphocytes. Again, light scatter analysis may reveal a range of cell sizes in the lymphoid population so that analysis can be focused on large and small cells separately. In our experience, the larger cells usually phenotype as the lymphoma/leukemia cells, whereas the smaller cells are residual small lymphocytes mixed in varying degree with small lymphoma cells. The example in Table 2 demonstrates that the B lymphoma phenotype is reflected most clearly in the large cell population where the great majority of cells phenotype as a clone of OKT10+, SIg (kappa)+, Ia+ cells. The OKT 10 antibody frequently binds to antigens on activated or proliferating T and B lymphocytes. The SIg clonality was apparent when all lymphoid cells were analyzed as one population, but there were obviously T cells present as well. Analysis of small lymphocytes alone may completely obscure clonality because of the mixture. This ability to focus on different subpopulations electronically is enhanced by appropriate computers which allow list mode data storage. Each cell signal is stored allowing recall

Table 2. Example: Percentage of Positive Cells in a Lymph Node Specimen from a 56-Year Old Female with a Diagnosis of B Cell Lymphoma.

Antibodies	All Lymphocytes	Large Lymphocytes
OKT 3	37	6
11	38	7
4	35	7
8	4	1
6	0	1
10	31	61
Anti-Ig (PV)	53	86
Anti-kappa	43	76
Anti-lambda	2	1
OKIa	50	96
cALLa	0	1
OKM_1	8	3

Table 3. Electronic Dissection of Flow Cytometric Data

Region of Cytogram	% of Total Cells in Gate	% Positive Cells Antibodies OKT 11	anti-Kappa	anti-Lambda
(large)				
1	3.5	2	88	17
2	2.5	2	87	14
3	0.9	1	89	16
4	7.0	6	85	10
5	9.6	10	86	9
6	16.5	19	78	14
7	36.5	24	69	13
8	23.5	25	70	12
9	0	--	--	--
(small)				

of cytograms so that different populations can be analyzed for each antibody in retrospect after the sample is gone. An example is seen in Table 3 in which the lymphoid cell cytogram has been "sliced" into nine population segments by calling up data for reanalysis. In this case B lymphoma cells are present in both large and small cell populations so that clonality is not obscured by T cells and normal residual B cells. In other cases the clonality may be obscured.

PreLymphomas. We have observed several cases over the past few years in which monoclonal SIg patterns were not associated with a histologic diagnosis of lymphoma or leukemia.[31] We considered technical errors or inadequate criteria for monoclonality, but concluded that these patients should be followed carefully. In view of recent findings that a significant number of patients with the persistent generalized lymphadenopathy (PGL) associated with the prodrome of AIDS have developed B cell lymphomas,[32-34] it appears that patients with reactive lymph node hyperplasia and monoclonal SIg patterns may well be in prelymphomatous phase of disease. In fact we have followed a patient who progressed from PGL to diagnostic lymphoma.

Recently, in reviewing a number of recent patients with B cell lymphoma of different cell types who had been studied for SIg clonality, we found that kappa/lambda ratios of less than 0.7 or greater than 5.5 identified lymphomas with only a 6% false-positive rate. Of more interest were those patients (4 of 49) who had histologically benign lymph nodes. Three of these four had PGL and the monoclonality in the fourth appeared to be due to a technical artifact.

The lesson to learn from such results is that phenotyping appears to offer a sensitive method for detecting patients who may have a high propensity for progressing to lymphoma. So far this applies to B cell lymphomas, where recognizing clonality is possible. If T cell neoplastic clonality can be recognized with new antibodies, the same predictiveness may be available for T cell lymphomas.

The Role of Immunoregulatory T Cells in Lymphoproliferative Disorders. There is increasing evidence that deficits in immunoregulation may play a role in the development of differentiation arrests associated with lymphocytic neoplasms, particularly in B-CLL.[35,36] Correction of these deficits in vitro has led to induced cell differentiation both morphologically and functionally. Because it is now possible to quantitate T cell subsets in B-lymphomas and leukemias, there has been interest in whether T cell subsets are altered, and if so, whether they play a role in such clinical features of B CLL as hypogammaglobulinemia.[37-40] We have observed significant differences in helper/suppressor ratios in small cleaved follicular center cell lymphomas as compared to lymph nodes showing reactive hyperplasia, but as yet have not determined their clinical or biological significance.

CONCLUSION

It is clear that flow cytometry and monoclonal antibodies are here to stay. They have been utilized primarily by investigators, but we are now at the stage of applying them in the clinical laboratory. It is important that pathologists and clinical physicians recognize this technology as having the potential for being extremely valuable, not only in phenotyping leucocytes in hematopoietic and immunologic disorders, but in application to other neoplastic processes. As monoclonal antibodies which recognize various tumor-associated antigens are made available, this technology can be applied to screening body fluids and tissue cell suspensions for neoplastic cells. Because of its sensitivity and the large numbers of cells analyzed in seconds, the approach should have great clinical utility in diagnosis and patient monitoring. Its value in monitoring posttransplantation patients for impending rejections is already apparent and a similar role in monitoring leukemia/lymphoma/cancer patients for the appearance of neoplastic cells in the blood or alterations in leucocyte populations which are involved in host defense is developing.

ACKNOWLEDGEMENTS

The studies described were done in collaboration with M. Hechinger, D. Boone, A. Levine, N. Levy, J. Louie, R. Lukes, and P. Meyer. Thanks go to Mrs. Linda Tedlock for manuscript preparation.

REFERENCES

1. Sachs L. 1982. Control of growth and normal differentiation in leukemic cells: Regulation of the development program and restoration of the normal phenotype in myeloid leukemia. J Cell Physiol (suppl) 1:151.
2. Greaves MF. 1982. Target cells, cellular phenotypes, and lineage fidelity in human leukemia. J Cell Physiol (suppl) 1:113.
3. Lukes RJ, Taylor CR, Parker JW, Lincoln TL, Pattengale PK and Tindle BH. 1978. A morphologic and immunologic surface marker study of 299 cases of non-Hodgkin's lymphomas and related leukemias. Am J Pathol 90:461-486.
4. Koehler G. and Milstein G. 1979. Continuous cultures of fused cells secreting antibody or predefined specificity. Nature 256:496.
5. Knowles DM, Dodson LD, Raab R, et al. 1983. The application of monoclonal antibodies to the characterization and diagnosis of lymphoid neoplasms: A review of recent studies. Diag Immunol 1:142-149.
6. Haynes BF, Eisenbath GS (eds). 1983. Monoclonal antibodies: Probes for the study of autoimmunity and immunodeficiency. New York, Academic Press.
7. Reinherz EL, Kung PC, Goldstein G, Levey RH, Schlossman SF. 1980. Discrete stages of human intrathymic differentiation: Analysis of normal thymocytes and leukemic lymphoblasts of T lineage. Proc Natl Acad Sci USA 77:1588-1592.
8. Keller RH, Milson TJ, Janicek KM, Patrick CW. 1984 (in press). Monoclonal antibodies: Clinical utility and the misunderstood epitope. Lab Med
9. Patrick CW, Milson TJ, McFadden PW, Keller RH. 1984 (in press). Flow cytometry and cell sorting: Important new clinical tools. Lab Med.
10. Hansen WP, Hoffman RA, Ip SH, Healey KW. 1982. Light scatter as an adjunct to cellular immunofluorescence in flow cytometry systems. J Clin Immunol (suppl) 2:325-415.
11. Ault KA. 1983. Clinical applications of fluorescence-activated cell sorting techniques. Diag Immunol 1:2-10.
12. LeBien TW, McKenna RW, Abramson CS, Gajl-Peczalska KJ, Nesbit ME, Coccia PF, Bloomfield CD, Brunning RD, Kersey JH. 1981. Use of monoclonal antibodies, morphology, and cytochemistry to probe the cellular heterogeneity of acute leukemia and lymphoma. Cancer Res 41:477-4780.
13. Foon KA, Schroff RW, Gale RP. 1982. Surface markers on leu-

kemia and lymphoma cells. Recent advances. Blood 60:1-19.
14. Greaves MF. 1981. Analysis of lymphoid phenotypes in acute leukemia: Their clinical and biological significances. Cancer Res 41:4752-4766.
15. Greaves MF. 1982. Target cells, cellular phenotypes and lineage fidelity in human leukemia. J Cell Physiol (supp) 1:113-125.
16. Zipf TF, Fox RI, Dilley J, Levy R. 1981. Definition of the high risk acute lymphoblastic leukemia patient by immunological phenotyping with monoclonal antibodies. Cancer Res 41:4786-4789.
17. Stass S, Merrs J, Melvin S, Peri C-H, Murphy SP, Williams P. 1984 (in press). Lineage switch in acute leukemia. Blood
18. Hershfield MS, Kurtzberg J, Harden E, Moore JO, Whang-Weng J, Haynes BF. 1984. Conversion of a stem cell leukemia from a T-lymphoid to a myeloid phenotype induced by adenosine deaminase inhibitor 2'-deoxycoformycin. Proc Natl Acad Sci USA 81:253.
19. Fialkow PJ, Singer JW, Adanison JW, Vaidja K, K.Dow LN, Ocha J, Moohr JW. 1981. Acute non-lymphocytic leukemia: heterogeneity of stem cell origin. Blood 301:144.
20. LeBien TW, Hozier J, Minowada J, Kersey JH. 1979. Origin of chronic myelocytic leukemia in a precursor of pre-B lymphocytes. New Engl J Med 301:144.
21. Bahhahi A, Minowada J, Arnold A, Cossman J, Jensen J, Wheng-Peng J, Waldman T, Korsmeyer S. 1983. Lymphoid blast crisis of chronic myelogenous leukemia represent stages in the development of B-cell precursors. New Engl J Med 309:826.
22. Rudders RA, Ahl ET Jr, DeLellis RA. 1981. Surface marker and histopathologic correlatin with long-term survival in advanced large-cell non-Hodgkin's lymphoma. Cancer 47:1329-1335.
23. Rudders RA, DeLellis RA, AHl ET, Bernstein S, Begg CB. 1982. Surface marker identificatin of small cleaved follicular center cell lymphomas with a highly favorable prognosis. Cancer Res 42:349-353.
24. Lukes RJ, Parker JW, Taylor CR, Tindle BH, Cramer AD, Lincoln TI. 1978. Immunological approach to non-Hodgkin's lymphomas and related leukemias. Analysis of the results of multiparameter studies of 425 cases. Semin Hematol 15:322-351.
25. Nadler LM, Stashenko P, Reinherz EL, Ritz J, Hardy R, Schlossman SF. 1982. Expression of normal differentiation antigens on human-leukemia and lymphoma cells. In: Malignant Lymphomas: Etiology, Immunology, Pathology, Treatment, SA Rosenberg,, HS Kaplan (eds). Academic Press, pp 107-120.
26. Greaves MF. 1982. Phenotypic diversity of T cell leukemias. J Clin Immunol (suppl 3) 2:75s-80s.
27. Jose DG, Pilkington GR, Wolf MM, Ding JC, van der Wegden MB, Gont T, Eng, Elliott P, Whiteside M. 1983. Diagnostic information derived from immunotyping 1000 patients with leukemia and lymphoma. Pathol 15:53-60.
28. Ault KA. 1979. Detection of small numbers of monoclonal B lymphocytes in the blood of patients with lymphoma. New Engl J Med 300:1401-1405.
29. Nagel JE, Chrest FJ, Pyle RS, Adler WH. 1983. Monoclonal antibody analysis of T lymphocyte subsets in young and aged adults. Immunol Commun 12:223-237.
30. Gascon P, Zanmbos NC, Young NS. 1984. Immunologic abnormalities in patients receiving multiple blood transfusions. Ann Int Med 100:173-177.

31. Levy N, Nelson J, Meyer P, Lukes RJ, Parker JW. 1983. Reactive lymphoid hyperplasia with single class (monoclonal) Surface immunoglobulin. Am J Clin Pathol 80:30-308.
32. Ziegler JL, Drew WL, Miner RC, et al. 1982. Outbreak of Burkitt's-like lymphoma in homosexual men. Lanset 2:631-633.
33. Levine AM, Meyer PR, Bergandy MK, Parker JW, Taylor CR, Irwin L, Lukes RJ. 1984. Development of B cell lymphoma in homosexual men: Clinical and immunologic findings. Ann Intern Med 100:7-13.
34. Ziegler JL, Beckstrad JA, Vlberling PA, et al. 1984. Non-Hodgkin's lymphoma in 90 homosexual men. Relationship to generalized lymphadenopathy and acquired immunodeficiency syndrome (AIDS). New Engl J Med 331:565-570.
35. Fu SM, Chiorazzi N, Kunkel HG, Halper JP, Harris SR. 1978. Induction of in vitro differentiation and immunoglobulin synthesis of human B lymphocytes. J Exp Med 148:1570-1578.
36. Yoshizski K, Nakagawa T, Kaieda T, Muraguchi A, Yamamura Y, Kishimoto T. 1982. Induction of proliferation and Ig production in human B leukemia cells by anti-immunoglobulins and T cell factors. J Immunol 128:1296-1301.
37. Barr IG, Toh BH. 1983. Routine flow cytometric diagnosis of lymphoproliferative disorders. J Clin Immunol 3:184-195.
38. Mills KH, Worman CP, Cawley JC. 1982. T cell subsets in chronic lymphocytic leukemia (CLL). Br J Haematol 50:710-712.
39. Platsoucas CD, Galinski M, et al. 1982. Abnormal T lymphocyte subpopulations in patients with B cell chronic lymphocytic leukemia: An analysis by monoclonal antibodies. J Immunol 129:2305-2312.
40. Matutes E, Wechsler A, et al. 1981. Unusual T cell phenotype in advanced B chronic lymphocytic leukemia. Br J Haematol 49:635-642.

CHANGING CONCEPTS IN THERAPY OF THE NON-HODGKIN LYMPHOMAS

SAUL A. ROSENBERG

INTRODUCTION

The management of patients with malignant lymphomas has undergone considerable change during the past ten years. As a result of advances in diagnostic and therapeutic methods, treatment results have dramatically improved for patients with Hodgkin's disease.[1,2] The situation is not the same for patients with lymphomas other than Hodgkin's disease, the so-called non-Hodgkin's lymphomas.[3]

Problems in this field are reflected by the continued proposals of new histopathologic classifications and nomenclature.[4-7] In part, this is due to new knowledge and concepts of the function of the lymphoid system. However, the search for new classifications and clinico-pathologic correlations is also motivated by the frustrations of managing these patients. The non-Hodgkin's lymphomas are a diverse group of diseases, varying from very aggressive and rapidly fatal to some of the most indolent and well-tolerated malignancies of man.

Children with lymphomas must be considered separately because they present quite different clinico-pathologic problems and require different management programs than for adults.[8]

Recommendations for management of patients with non-Hodgkin's lymphomas are made more difficult, not only by changing nomenclature, but also by problems in defining histologic subgroups, variable diagnostic criteria of investigators reporting treatment results, reporting of benefit of treatment results in terms of remission rather than survival changes, and the general lack of well-controlled clinical trials in this field of study.

Yet these diseases are relatively common, and physicians must select management methods based upon currently available evidence and experience.

CLASSIFICATION RECOMMENDATIONS

There are at least six major classification systems for the non-Hodgkin's lymphomas. The situation is further complicated because of continual modifications of the classifications by their proponents and the limited clinico-pathologic correlations supporting each proposal.

At this time, a modified Rappaport classification is a very useful system for clinicians. It is relatively well understood and utilized by clinicians and pathologists. This and other systems can be utilized to separate patients into those of good, or favorable, types; poor, or unfavorable, types; and a third group, those with lymphoblastic lymphomas (convoluted or non-convoluted types). For the purpose of this discussion, the modified Rappaport system will be used.

MANAGEMENT CONSIDERATIONS OTHER THAN PATHOLOGIC GROUP

There are very important variables and considerations which must be used in arriving at management decisions other than the histologic subtype. These are:

(1) the extent of the disease, or stage of the patient[9]
(2) the site or sites of involvement
(3) the size or mass of the tumor in various sites
(4) the symptoms of the patient, both local and systemic
(5) the threat of serious problems, ie, ureteral obstruction, airway compromise, meningeal involvement
(6) bone marrow function
(7) the age of the patient
(8) the variable of time, or the "tempo" of the patient's tumor progression

Also to be considered in selecting a treatment program are the experience and facilities available to the physician and whether or not the patient, with informed consent, is willing to participate in a clinical trial.

DIAGNOSTIC STUDIES

Management decisions for patients with lymphomas should not be made until the extent of the disease is determined, within the limitations of our currently available methods.

It is axiomatic that all patients should have a careful history and physical examination. In addition to routine blood counts and screening chemistries, the bone marrow should be evaluated for involvement by an adequate biopsy, usually of the posterior iliac crest. Paradoxically, bone marrow involvement will be found frequently in patients in the lymphocytic group, who have good prognoses, and infrequently in the histiocytic group. One adequate needle biopsy, with the Jamshidi needle, is usually sufficient. Additional biopsies will improve the yield[10] and should be obtained if the initial biopsy is inadequate or scanty or, in a patient in the lymphocytic group, if the demonstration of bone marrow involvement would change the management recommendation.

The lower extremity lymphogram is important to obtain in all patients in whom there is no specific contraindication (i.e., serious cardiopulmonary disease). The opacified retroperitoneal lymph nodes, whether normal or abnormal, can be valuable indicators of the tempo of the disease and can indicate progression or regression during and after the completion of treatment programs. There may be abnormal abdominal lymph nodes, especially in the mesentery, which are not seen on the lymphogram. These may be better demonstrated by computerized axial tomography or laparotomy, but the ease of making sequential comparative examinations after lymphography by subsequent plain abdominal roentgengram makes the lymphogram an indicated and valuable procedure.

The use of diagnostic laparotomy should be much more restricted for patients with non-Hodgkin's lymphomas than for those with Hodgkin's disease. It is recommended primarily for the patient under 50 years of age with favorable lymphoma, who after bone marrow biopsy and lymphography, has clinical stages I or II disease (according to the Ann Arbor classification). Its primary purpose is to demonstrate stage III or IV disease, situations in which radiation therapy is not recommended; whereas it is for those with localized disease. Exploratory laparotomy is not usually indicated for patients with unfavorable lymphomas. The yield in finding occult disease is low, especially in those under 40.[11] A significant number of patients in the poorer prognostic group will have their disease discovered at laparotomy, and a second procedure is usually not indicated to clarify the extent of intra-abdominal disease.

Isotope scans to evaluate the bones, liver and spleen, or gallium scans, have limited usefulness in this group of diseases. They should not be considered diagnostic, and other radiologic or biopsy methods should be used to establish sites of involvement which would change the management recommendation.

MANAGEMENT RECOMMENDATIONS

Favorable Prognostic Group

Patients with favorable type lymphomas of stage I and II extent are uncommon. However, approximately 10% of patients will have localized disease even after extensive diagnostic evaluation, including laparotomy. Radiation therapy to the involved sites is indicated. These are very radiosensitive tumors and local control of the disease may result for many years. No controlled trial clarifies the extent of irradiation that should be used.[3] Cures should not be concluded for these patients, even if disease recurrence is not seen for five to ten years. The disease may be so indolent and well tolerated that clinical recurrence may not be evident for many years.

Patients with favorable lymphomas of stage III and IV extent are probably not curable by any known therapy program. This has been true despite the observation that these patients are highly responsive to a variety of treatment programs, including combination chemotherapy, radiation therapy, or both. Despite documented remission, the disease usually recurs at a rate of about 10%-15% per year, for a period of 10 years or longer after treatment completion.[12] The only exception to this observation has been a small group of patients with nodular mixed lymphoma treated at the National Cancer Institute (NCI), with the C-MOPP (cyclophosphamide, vincristine, procarbazine, and prednisone) program.[13] This group has reported a low risk of recurrence after complete remission. These results have not yet been confirmed by others.

It is therefore recommended that a palliative treatment approach should be adopted for patients with favorable lymphomas of stage III and IV extent. In some patients, no initial treatment is required if they are asymptomatic, and the size or location of the lymphadenopathy poses no major threat.[14] Much can be learned in these patients, who are usually over the age of 50, by observing their status and lymph node size over a period of months before recommending a treatment program. Some will be stable over many months, even years, and treatment can be delayed. For a few, especially the elderly, it may never be required. Some will have spontaneous regressions, usually with subsequent recurrences. For other patients, within the first year and, in time, for most patients, the lymph nodes will gradually enlarge. If the rate of growth is rapid, i.e., over a few months, and if systemic symptoms are noted, combination chemotherapy with a regimen employing cyclophosphamide, vincristine, and prednisone is advised. The so-called CVP regimen of the NCI is a good one.[15] The drugs are usually given in cycles until a complete remission is obtained, by all studies available, and then discontinued. If the disease progresses slowly over a period of many months, or the patient is anxious because of the appearance of the lymphadenopathy, continuous or intermittent oral single agent alkylating agent therapy can be satisfactory. Chlorambucil is a well-tolerated drug for this purpose. A dose of 6-12 mg/day is usually given until good disease regression is noted. A daily dose may then be reduced or given bimonthly at 20-40 mg per dose, monitoring peripheral blood counts, or may be discontinued.

Local irradiation for major bulky sites of disease should always be considered in the palliative program for these patients, especially for ureteral obstruction, lower extremity edema, mediastinal masses, chylous effusions with paravertebral masses and cosmetic problems.

Low dose whole body irradiation[16,17] is an acceptable alternative to systemic chemotherapy for patients with stage III and IV disease, provided they have not been treated extensively with prior chemotherapy, platelet counts are adequate, and radiotherapists experienced with the technique are available.

A challenging problem is the occasional younger patient, in the 20 to 40 year old range, who has stage III or IV favorable lymphoma. Despite the relatively good prognosis, the patient's life will probably be shortened by the disease. It is tempting and understandable for physicians to recommend aggressive treatment for younger patients with these very responsive lymphomas. Complete remissions are often obtained. Yet, no survival benefit is available to support this approach. The physician and patient should acknowledge this fact before proceeding.

Unfavorable Lymphoma

Despite the overall poorer prognoses of this group of patients, the clinical problems and responses to therapy are quite variable. Paradoxically, prolonged disease-free survival is more often possible and demonstrable for this group of patients than for the "favorable" group, despite their poorer natural history. An active treatment program is always indicated, no matter how limited the disease, how asymptomatic the patient, or, at the other extreme, how widespread the tumor or how critically ill the patient.

A high proportion of patients with stage I and I_E disease, diffuse histiocytic lymphoma, limited to a single lymph node region or an isolated extranodal site, may be cured of their disease by surgery and/or radiotherapy. In some patients who present with gastrointestinal tumor, surgery has been required to establish the diagnosis. Radical surgical procedures and lymph node dissections should not be performed, but radiation therapy in adequate doses should be used to control the primary tumor and regional lymph node areas. If careful staging methods are employed, patients with stage I and I_E disease can be cured in approximately 75% of the cases.[18].

Patients with stage II and II_E disease are more difficult to manage. Despite careful evaluation and staging, only 25%-40% are permanently controlled by surgery and/or radiation therapy. It is recommended that combined modality programs be used for these patients in a sequence which is best individualized to a particular clinical setting and problem. Surgery may be necessary to establish the diagnosis, and radiotherapy may be very effective in reducing large tumor masses. However, combination chemotherapy, such as C-MOPP regimen of NCI,[13] or the CHOP (cyclophosphamide, adriamycin, vincristine, and prednisone) regimen of the Southwest Oncology Group[19] should improve the cure rates of these patients. Clinical trials have not yet established this point, however.

Patients with stage III and IV unfavorable lymphomas should all receive combination chemotherapy. Despite widespread disease and an unfavorable natural history, prolonged disease-free survival and probable cure is possible to achieve in a significant proportion of these patients.[13] Those with disease limited to lymph nodes, or stage III extent, have the best chemotherapy results and more than 50% can be cured with the chemotherapy programs. Those with stage

IV disease, especially with bone marrow involvement, do not fare as well, probably less than 25% being controlled for long periods. The role of radiation therapy in these patients with stages III and IV disease is not established.

It may be that within the diverse group of patients with unfavorable lymphomas, as grouped in this discussion, there are different clinical entities which should have different treatment approaches and prognoses. There is some evidence that the newer classifications and immunologic-morphologic techniques can help identify these subgroups.[20-22] However, we must await more information before patients can be selected within this poorer prognostic category for different management programs.

Lymphoblastic Lymphomas

An important clinico-pathologic entity has been recognized by Lukes and others which had been previously included in the diffuse lymphomas, poorly differentiated lymphocytic type of Rappaport.[23,24]

These patients are rare, but have distinctive clinical features. The disease occurs in younger individuals, often presenting with large mediastinal masses. The disease merges clinically and morphologically with acute lymphoblastic leukemia of poor prognosis. Despite initial drug and radiosensitive, recurrent and subsequent involvement of the bone marrow and meninges is common, with a rapidly fatal course.

Systemic chemotherapy programs of the types used for unfavorable childhood acute leukemia[25,26] or for adult lymphoblastic leukemia are indicated, no matter how localized the lymphoblastic lymphoma appears to be. Central nervous system prophylaxis employing intrathecal methotrexate and cranial irradiation, or a comparable program, is required to prevent meningeal relapse. The St. Judes' program for unfavorable childhood acute leukemia[24] is an acceptable one, although there is inadequate data to compare different regimens at this time.

REFERENCES

1. Kaplan HS. 1972. Hodgkin's disease. Cambridge, Mass. Harvard University Press.
2. DeVita VT Jr, Lewis BJ, Rozencweig M, et al. 1978. The chemotherapy of Hodgkin's disease: past experiences and future directions. Cancer 42:979-990.

3. Glatstein E, Donaldson SS, Rosenberg SA, et al. 1977. Combined mortality therapy in malignant lymphomas. Cancer Treat Rep 61:1199-1208.
4. Lukes RJ, Collins RD. 1977. Lukes-Collins classification and its significance. Cancer Treat Rep 61:971-979.
5. Lennert K, Mohri N, Stein H, et al. 1975. The histopathology of malignant lymphoma. Br J Haematol 31(Suppl):193-203.
6. Dorfman RF. 1977. Pathology of the non-Hodgkin's lymphomas: new classifications. Cancer Treat Rep 61:945-951.
7. Bennett MH, Farrer-Brown G, Henry K, et al. 1974. Classification of non-Hodgkin's lymphomas. Lancet 2:405-406.
8. Murphy SB. 1978. Current concepts in cancer: childhood non-Hodgkin's lymphoma. New Engl J Med 299:1446-1448.
9. Carbone PP, Kaplan HS, Musshoff K, et al. 1971. Report of the committee of Hodgkin's disease staging classification. Cancer Res 31:1860-1861.
10. Brunning RD, Bloomfield CD, McKenna RW, et al. 1975. Bilateral trephine bone marrow biopsies in lymphoma and other neoplastic diseases. Ann Intern Med 82:365-366.
11. Goffinet DR, Warnke R, Dunnick NR, et al. 1977. Clinical and surgical (laparotomy) evaluation of patients with non-Hodgkin's lymphomas. Cancer Treat Rep 61:981-992.
12. Portlock CS, Rosenberg SA, Glatstein E, et al. 1976. Treatment of advanced non-Hodgkin's lymphomas with favorable histologies: preliminary results of a prospective trial. Blood 47:747-756.
13. Anderson T, Bender RA, Fisher RI, et al. 1977. Combination chemotherapy in non-Hodgkin's lymphoma: results of long-term followup. Cancer Treat Rep 61:1057-1066.
14. Portlock CS, Rosenberg SA. 1977. Chemotherapy of the non-Hodgkin's lymphomas: the Stanford experience. Cancer Treat Rep 61:1049-1055.
15. Bagley CM Jr, DeVita VT, Berard CW, et al. 1972. Advanced lymphosarcoma: intensive cyclical combination chemotherapy with cyclophosphamide, vincristine, and prednisone. Ann Intern Med 76:227-234.
16. Chaffey JT, Hellman S, Rosenthal DS, et al. 1977. Total-body irradiation in the treatment of lymphocytic lymphoma. Cancer Treat Rep 61:1149-1152.
17. Young RC, Johnson RE, Canellos GP, et al. 1977. Advanced lymphocytic lymphoma: randomized comparisons of chemotherapy and radiotherapy, alone or in combination. Cancer Treat Rep 61:1153-1159.
18. Bush RS, Gospodarowicz M, Sturgeon J, et al. 1977. Radiation therapy of localized non-Hodgkin's lymphoma. Cancer Treat Rep 61:1129-1136.
19. McKelvey EM, Gottlieb JA, Wilson HE, et al. 1976. Hydroxyldaunomycin (adriamycin) combination chemotherapy in malignant lymphoma. Cancer 38:1484-1493.
20. Strauchen JA, Young RC, DeVita VT, et al. 1978. Clinical relevance of the histopathological subclassification of diffuse histiocytic lymphoma. New Engl J Med 299:1382-1387.
21. Bloomfield CD, Kersey JH, Brunning RD, et al. 1976. Prognostic significance of lymphocyte surface markers in adult non-Hodgkin's malignant lymphoma. Lancet 2:1330-1333.
22. Lukes RJ, Taylor CR, Parker JW, et al. 1978. A morphologic and immunologic surface marker study of 299 cases of non-Hodgkin lymphomas and related leukemias. Am J Pathol 90:461-486.

23. Nathwani BN, Kim H, Rappaport H. 1976. Malignant lymphoma, lymphoblastic. Cancer 38:964-983.
24. Barcos MP, Lukes RJ. 1975. Malignant lymphoma of convoluted lymphocytes: A new entity of possible T-cell type. In: Conflicts in Childhood Cancer. Progress in Clinical and Biological Research, Vol 4. New York, Alan R Liss Inc, pp 147-178.
25. Murphy SB. 1977. Management of childhood non-Hodgkin's disease. Cancer Treat Rep 61:1161-1173.
26. Weinstein HJ, Vance ZB, Jeffe N, et al. 1979. Improved prognosis for patients with mediastinal lymphoblastic lymphoma. Blood 53:687-694.

BIOLOGICAL APPROACHES TO THE THERAPY OF LYMPHOPROLIFERATIVE DISEASES

KENNETH A. FOON

1. INTRODUCTION

Progress has been made over the past 5 years toward the development of specific biological approaches to the treatment of cancer. The techniques of genetic engineering and mass cell culture and improved techniques in protein and nucleic acid sequencing have made available biologics as highly purified molecules. The most definitive investigations have been carried out with the various interferon (IFN) preparations, and it is clear that they are capable of inducing responses primarily in patients with certain types of lymphomas and leukemias. Recent monoclonal antibody data, while interesting, have not yet demonstrated that monoclonal antibodies are effective in the treatment of lymphoma/leukemia. Intensive investigations are currently under way in both of these areas of clinical research.

2. INTERFERON

IFNs are a family of proteins produced by cells in response to virus, double-stranded ribonucleic acid, antigens, and mitogens. In addition to antiviral activity, the IFNs have profound effects on the immune system. IFNs have direct anti-proliferative activity; can alter expression of cell surface antigens; and can influence a number of components of the immune system, including B, T, and natural killer cells and macrophages. With respect to the IFNs and cancer therapy, it is still unclear whether the IFNs work primarily by their antiproliferative activity or through alterations of immune responses. It is clear, however, from both the preclinical and clinical studies that IFNs have antitumor activity in a number of tumor systems.

IFNs are currently classified according to various biochemical properties into three groups designated as IFN-α, IFN-β, and IFN-γ. IFN-α and IFN-β (previously grouped together as type I interferons) are acid stable and are produced primarily by leukocytes and fibroblasts, respectively, in response to viruses or double-stranded ribonucleic acid. Lymphoblastic cells produce a mixture of type I interferon consisting of approximately 90% IFN-α and 10% IFN-β. In contrast, IFN-γ (type II interferon) is an acid-stable IFN produced by T lymphocytes and large granular lymphocytes in response to mitogen or antigen exposure and is often referred to as immune IFN.

The most extensively clinically studied interferons are the natural and recombinant IFN-α preparations. Major activity appears to be primarily in lymphoproliferative disorders including non-Hodgkin's lymphomas (NHL) (1-4) and hairy cell leukemia (5). At the National Cancer Institute we recently completed a phase II IFN trial for previously treated patients with NHL, chronic lymphocytic leukemia (CLL), and cutaneous T-cell lymphoma (CTCL or mycosis fungoides). Dr. Paul Bunn of the NCI-Navy Oncology Branch was the principal investigator of the CTCL arm of the study. Patients were treated with recombinant leukocyte A interferon (rIFN-αA, Hoffman-La Roche, Nutley, N.J.) at 50 x 10^6 U/m^2 body surface area three times weekly by the intramuscular route. The dose and schedule were designed based on the maximum tolerated dose from our phase I study with rIFN-αA (4). Patients were treated for 3 months, and dose reductions to 50% and then 10% of the starting dose were made based on unacceptable toxicity (e.g., fatigue, anorexia, leukopenia, elevated hepatic transaminases).

Eighty-four patients were entered on our phase II lymphoma/leukemia trial. Forty-five of these patients had NHL (6), 19 had CLL (7), and 30 had CTCL (8). Major toxic reactions observed were fever, chills, fatigue, and anorexia. The average duration of therapy at 100% dosage was 2.5 weeks and 6.5 weeks at 50% dose. Fatigue was the most common reason for dose reduction.

Our results indicate significant antitumor activity for rIFN-αA in patients with low grade and intermediate grade histology NHL classified by the Working Formulation (9), as well as in patients with CTCL (Table 1). There was little evidence of activity for CLL; in fact, 11 of 18 evaluable patients with CLL progressed while on rIFN-αA therapy (7). Fifty percent of the patients with low grade and intermediate grade histology NHL (6) and nearly 50% with CTCL responded with either partial or complete responses (8). All responding patients were maintained on rIFN-αA therapy; the median duration of response is 8 months for NHL and 7 months for CTCL. The five complete responders with low grade and intermediate grade histology NHL were shown to be tumor free in sites of previous disease by noninvasive studies and biopsies where indicated. The responses in patients with CTCL included reductions of the size of skin plaques and tumors, lymph nodes, and circulating Sézary cells. It was particularly interesting that all of the responding patients had very advanced disease and had failed multiple courses of combination chemotherapy.

Table 1. Clinical responses in the National Cancer Institute phase II recombinant leukocyte A interferon trials for lymphoproliferative disorders.

Disease*	Evaluable patients	Complete response	Partial response	Minimal or no response	Progression
Low grade NHL	24	4	9	7	4
Intermediate grade NHL	6	1	1	1	3
High grade NHL	7	0	1	1	5
CLL	18	0	2	5	11
CTCL	19	0	9	7	3
HCL	7	0	6	1	0

*NHL, non-Hodgkin's lymphoma; CLL, chronic lymphocytic leukemia; CTCL, cutaneous T cell lymphoma; HCL, hairy cell leukemia.

We have recently begun a phase II trial of rIFN-αA for hairy cell leukemia patients based on the excellent results using natural IFN-α reported by Quesada and co-workers (5). Seven patients were treated with intramuscular and/or subcutaneous injections of rIFN-αA at 3 x 10^6 U daily and have completed at least 8 weeks of treatment. Six patients have responded with substantial improvement in their hematologic parameters. The only major toxicity was transient myelosuppression during the first week of therapy. Preliminary immunologic results have demonstrated improvement in natural killer activity and normalization of lymphoid subpopulations, coincident with improved hematologic parameters.

3. CONCLUSION FROM IFN-α TRIALS

Our phase II studies have demonstrated that rIFN-αA has the highest reported response rate for any standard or experimental agent in advanced previously treated CTCL patients. It also establishes rIFN-αA as a new non-cross-resistant modality of therapy in low grade and intermediate grade histology NHL. Finally, we have confirmed earlier reports that α-IFN is the most active single agent for hairy cell leukemia and should be considered for therapy when splenectomy is no longer effective in controlling the disease. Phase III trials in previously untreated NHL, CTCL, and hairy cell leukemia patients are clear avenues of future investigation.

4. CLINICAL EVALUATION OF MONOCLONAL ANTIBODIES

Monoclonal antibody therapy in humans has recently been reviewed (10-12). While most of these trials involved individual patients or very small series of patients, early indications are that monoclonal antibody alone may have some therapeutic effect in certain human malignancies, albeit rather limited. Most of these early trials have been designed to approach preliminary questions with respect to the feasibility and toxicity of monoclonal antibody therapy and the rationale for the use of these reagents (Table 2).

Table 2. Monoclonal antibody clinical trials for lymphoproliferative disorders.

Institution	Disease*	Antibody/Class	Specificity	No. of patients	Toxicity	Effect	Reference
Dana Farber	B-lymphoma	Ab89/IgG_{2a}	Lymphoma	1	Renal (transient)	Transient reduction in circulating cells	14
Dana Farber	cALL	J5/IgG_{2a}	CALLA	4	Fever (101-102°F)	Transient reduction in circulating cells	13
Stanford	T-CLL	L17F12 (anti-Leu-1)/IgG_{2a}	Leu-1	1	Renal, hepatic (transient)	Transient reduction in circulating cells	19
Stanford	CTCL	L17F12/IgG_{2a}	Leu-1	6	Dyspnea, hives, cutaneous pain	Minor remission in 5 of 7 patients	20
Stanford	B-lymphoma	4D6/IgG_{2a}	Idiotype	1	None	Complete remission 24+ months	23
Stanford	B-lymphoma		Idiotype	7	Fever, chills, nausea, vomitting, dyspnea, headache, diarrhea	4 of 7 partial remissions	24
U. Calif. San Diego	B-CLL	T101/IgG_{2a}	T65	4	Dyspnea, hypotension, fever, malaise, urticaria	Transient reduction in circulating cells	15,16
U. Calif. San Diego	CTCL	T101/IgG_{2a}	T65	4	Dyspnea, fever	Minor remissions	16
NCI	B-CLL	T101/IgG_{2a}	T65	13	Dyspnea, fever, hypotension, fever (101-102°F)	Transient reduction in circulating cells	17
NCI	CTCL	T101/IgG_{2a}	T65	12	Dyspnea, fever, (101-102°F)	Minor remission in 4 of 8 patients	21

*cALL, common acute lymphoblastic leukemia; T-CLL, T-chronic lymphocytic leukemia; CTCL, cutaneous T cell lymphoma.

5. ACUTE LYMPHOBLASTIC LEUKEMIA

Four patients with acute lymphoblastic leukemia were treated with escalating doses of the J5 monoclonal antibody, which binds to the common acute lymphoblastic leukemia antigen (CALLA) (13). In this study, patients demonstrated transient reductions in the circulating leukemia cells immediately following therapy with J5 antibody, and they demonstrated in vivo antibody localization to circulating and bone marrow tumor cells. Anti-murine antibody responses were not described; however, resistance to therapy was mediated in part by antigenic modulation of CALLA (loss of antigen from the cell surface membrane) in response to treatment with J5 antibody.

6. NON-HODGKIN'S LYMPHOMA AND CHRONIC LYMPHOCYTIC LEUKEMIA

The first monoclonal antibody therapy trial was reported by Nadler et al. (14). In this study, a patient with B-cell-derived lymphoma was treated with Ab89 in increasing dosages up to 1500 mg infused intravenously over 6 hours. There was a transient reduction in circulating tumor cells as well as a transient drop in creatinine clearance. A number of patients with B-cell-derived CLL have been treated at the University of California, San Diego, and at the National Cancer Institute (15-17) with the T101 antibody that recognizes a 65,000 to 67,000 molecular weight glycoprotein designated the T65 antigen. Patients in these studies have been treated with total dosages ranging from 8 to 400 mg (single doses ranging from 1 to 140 mg). Transient reductions in circulating leukemia cell counts were described in most of these patients; however, in only 2 patients was there a sustained reduction of 50% of the total circulating leukemia cells throughout the 4 weeks of therapy (17). However, even in those 2 patients, the levels rose to above baseline following the completion of the antibody therapy. There were no responses in lymph nodes or organs in any of these patients. As most of these patients were stage IV by the Rai classification and were hypogammaglobulinemic, it was not surprising that they were unable to mount anti-murine antibody responses.

A number of groups have treated patients with CTCL with either the T101 monoclonal antibody or the anti-Leu-1 monoclonal antibody, both of which react with the same glycoprotein (18-21). In these studies, a number of patients demonstrated transient improvements in their cutaneous skin lesions, and in some cases, there was shrinkage of enlarged lymph nodes. Because these patients were generally immunocompetent, a number of them mounted anti-murine antibody responses.

A more specific approach to the use of monoclonal therapy is the use of anti-idiotype monoclonal antibodies. Immunoglobulin molecules have a unique region in their variable portion, termed the "idiotype." The idiotype for every immunoglobulin molecule is different. As B-cell diseases are clonal diseases, each tumor cell expressed the same immunoglobulin molecule; therefore, the idiotype is identical on every tumor cell. In this unique situation, the idiotype is therefore a tumor-specific antigen. A group of investigators from Stanford developed a monoclonal antibody to the idiotypic determinant from a patient with a B-cell lymphoma who had become resistant to cytotoxic drugs and IFN (22). This patient was treated with eight dosages of anti-idiotype monoclonal antibody intravenously in a dose-escalation fashion, and he eventually entered a complete remission that has persisted for over 2 years (23). Seven additional patients have been treated, with only four partial remissions lasting from 1 to 6 months (24). Our first patient treated with an anti-idiotype monoclonal antibody at the National Cancer Institute had CLL and bulky lymphadenopathy. He was treated sequentially with first an IgG_{2b} antibody and then an IgG_1 antibody to a total dose of 2 grams of antibody. There was no response, due to circulating idiotype (50 μg/ml), which prevented binding of antibody to tumor cells. We were unable to control this despite extensive plasmapheresis.

A number of problems must be addressed with regard to anti-idiotype therapy. Developing anti-idiotype antibody is a labor-intensive project and may not be practical on a large scale. It is hoped that this process can be refined as new technology is developed. In addition, anti-idiotype antibodies are patient specific and, therefore, can be used to treat only a single patient. Two additional problems have recently been identified which will also limit the therapeutic role for anti-idiotype antibody in certain patients. First, some tumors are biclonal and would require more than one antibody for successful therapy (25). Second, the idiotype may be unstable on some patients' tumor cells likely due to somatic mutation within the variable region gene (26).

7. TOXICITY WITH UNCONJUGATED ANTIBODIES

Toxicities associated with monoclonal antibody therapy are generally quite mild. One problem witnessed in the National Cancer Institute clinical trial with T101 was shortness of breath and chest tightness either during or immediately following a 2-hour infusion of T101 at dosages of 50 mg or greater (17,21). While this toxicity was transient with no residual side effects, patients were extremely uncomfortable, and we were forced to stop therapy in a number of patients. In one instance, a patient developed perfusion abnormalities on a lung scan, and in another case, a patient developed a pulmonary infiltrate, both coincident with shortness of breath and resolved within 1 or 2 weeks. It was hypothesized that the rapid infusion of a large quantity of antibody resulted in binding to circulating cells, followed by leukoagglutination with micropulmonary emboli. It did not appear to be an anaphylactic reaction, as there was no response to epinephrine or measurable antigen-specific IgE levels. Furthermore, some of the patients experiencing pulmonary toxicity were subsequently treated with prolonged infusions of the same antibody without recurrence of these symptoms. In addition, patients treated with rapid infusions of much greater dosages of the 9.2.27 antimelanoma monoclonal antibody (500 mg), which does not bind to any circulating cells, never developed this toxicity. We have completely eliminated this toxicity with T101 by infusing the antibody at rates slower than 5 mg/hr.

Rare patients have developed hypotension and tachycardia following the infusion of murine monoclonal antibody (15,17). Urticaria has been a common problem,has rapidly responded to antihistamines, and has not prevented subsequent therapies. Fever, chills, flushing, nausea, and vomiting have been reported but have generally been minor problems. Occasional patients have developed a transient reduction in their creatinine clearance and an elevation of their liver enzymes (14,17). These were thought to be secondary to immune complexes between monoclonal antibody and circulating antigen. We have also witnessed two cases of a serum sickness-like syndrome in patients treated on our 9.2.27 antimelanoma monoclonal antibody protocol (27). In conclusion, murine-derived monoclonal antibodies can be safely infused, although side effects can be expected and they are usually mild.

8. OBSTACLES TO SUCCESSFUL THERAPY WITH UNCONJUGATED ANTIBODIES

One major problem with monoclonal antibody therapy is antigenic modulation, leading to loss of antigen from the cell surface membrane within minutes to hours after exposure to antibody (Table 3). The modulated cells will usually reexpress the antigen within 24 to 36 hours after the antibody infusion has been completed (when residual antibody is no longer in the serum). During the time that the cells are modulated, they no longer bind to the antibody. Not all antibody-antigen systems appear to modulate the antigen from the cell surface membrane. For instance, we have seen rapid and complete modulation of the T65 antigen following T101 therapy; however, we have not witnessed modulation of the 250,000 molecular weight glycoprotein/proteoglycan recognized by the 9.2.27 antimelanoma monoclonal antibody. While modulation may be a limiting problem for unconjugated free antibody, it may be an important positive factor for immunoconjugates. The antitumor effect of immunoconjugates may be dependent on modulation and internalization of the immunoconjugate-antigen complex. We have demonstrated that the T101-T65 complex is internalized at least 50%, which might make it an ideal antibody for drug and toxin conjugates (28).

Murine-derived monoclonal antibodies can stimulate the development of human antibodies to the murine immunoglobulin. This has been a limiting factor in some of the therapies with monoclonal antibodies, particularly in patients who are immuno-

Table 3. Therapeutic problems with monoclonal antibody therapy.

Problems	Possible solutions
Antigenic modulation	Choose monoclonal antibodies that recognize antigens that do not modulate. Conjugate drugs and toxins to antibodies.
Anti-mouse antibodies	Human antibodies, immunosuppressive drugs, plasmapheresis with immunospecific absorption, large dose of antibody to induce tolerance
Tumor heterogeneity	Treat with multiple antibodies that react with different antigens.
Neoplastic cells outside blood supply	Conjugate monoclonal antibody to radionuclides that "emit" radiation beyond a single cell.
Lack of in vivo cytotoxicity of antibody	Conjugate monoclonal antibody to drugs, toxins, or radionuclides.

logically intact. In our own studies, none of the patients with CLL developed anti-murine antibodies, while most of the patients with CTCL and one third of the patients with melanoma developed anti-murine antibodies (29). We detected the anti-murine response directed toward the idiotype of the 9.2.27 antibody in only 1 patient, and this was the only patient in whom it appeared that anti-mouse antibodies limited the ability of antibody to bind to tumor cells in vivo. Sears et al. (30) reported that 8 of 9 patients who received less than 200 mg of murine antibody developed anti-murine antibody, while only 1 of 9 patients who received over 366 mg developed antibodies, suggesting the high dose led to tolerance. A number of approaches might be useful in overcoming the problem of human anti-mouse responses. Human-derived monoclonal antibodies would eliminate this problem, although antiglobulin responses to the idiotype of the human immunoglobulin would still be possible. Low-dose cyclophosphamide given with the initial antibody infusion to destroy the clones producing the antiglobulin might be effective. Finally, infusing high doses of antibody (> 400 mg) at the onset of therapy might induce tolerance, as suggested by Sears and co-workers (30).

A problem with some antibody-tumor systems is tumor heterogeneity, with only a portion of the tumor cells reacting with a single antibody. This might be overcome by using multiple monoclonal antibodies reacting with different antigenic determinants. However, it should also be emphasized that the dividing tumor stem cell will be the critical cell to eliminate in any successful monoclonal antibody therapy. It is possible that a specific antigen may be expressed on all of the tumor stem cells, yet its expression is heterogeneous on the majority of tumor cells. Thus, the tumor could theoretically be cured by a single antibody (immunoconjugate) that does not bind to all of the tumor cells but does bind to all of the tumor stem cells.

Another problem is that the blood supply of tumor cells may be poor and, therefore, the antibody may not localize well on the tumor cells. This problem may in part be overcome by conjugating antibodies to radioisotopes that emit α particles. In this way, elimination of tumor cells may not be dependent on antibody binding to every tumor cell given the "field effect" of radiation.

Finally, monoclonal antibodies do not appear to be very effective in eliminating tumor cells by themselves (perhaps with the exception of antiidiotype antibody). Possibly if antibodies are conjugated to drug, toxins, or radioisotopes, more cytotoxic reagents capable of a greater antitumor effect can be developed. This is a major direction of our current research and is addressed in depth below.

9. CLINICAL TRIALS WITH IMMUNOCONJUGATES

A considerable body of evidence suggests, at least in animal tumor models, that antibodies covalently linked to certain toxins, such as ricin or diphtheria toxin, and certain drugs, such as doxorubicin, have a greater antitumor effect both in vitro and in vivo than do unconjugated free antibodies (31). A number of centers are studying toxin and drug conjugates with murine antibodies directed toward human malignancies, but none has of yet been taken into clinical trials.

Clinical trials using antisera or monoclonal antibodies conjugated to radionuclides primarily for tumor imaging have been widely performed. Most of these trials have been for patients with solid tumors and will be briefly reviewed as they are relevant to our own imaging trials for lymphoma. This subject has recently been reviewed by Goldenberg and DeLand (32). Goldenberg and co-workers conjugated ^{131}iodine by the chloramine-T method to anti-CEA immunoglobulins (heteroantisera). In order to compensate for background radioactivity, ^{99m}Tc pertechnetate and serum albumin were injected before imaging with ^{131}iodine anti-CEA (33). The ^{99m}Tc radioactivity was subtracted from that of the ^{131}I. They have used these methods of radioimmunodetection in over 450 patients using antibodies against a variety of hormones. They have seen no untoward effects in these subjects who have received multiple injections of the radioantibodies and they appear to have a high sensitivity for selectively detecting tumors. For instance, in colorectal cancer, they have shown a 91% overall true positive rate of cancer detection and localization for both primary and metastatic sites. They have also determined retrospectively that in 11 of 51 colorectal cancer patients, tumors not revealed by other methods of detection were disclosed by their radioimmunodetection. The cause of failure to image a tumor was due to the presence of a lesion less than 2 cm in diameter or a malignancy that was devoid of CEA. In similar studies reported by Mach and co-workers (34), positive scans were obtained in only 41% of patients with CEA-producing tumors.

One interesting observation was the inability of circulating CEA antigen to block the anti-CEA-antibody localization to tumors. In many of these patients, there were high levels of circulating CEA, yet excellent scanning was noted. This was possibly due to a higher affinity of the antibody for the antigen that is cell bound than the free circulating antigen. In some cases, there was evidence for the presence of complexes between circulating CEA and radioactive immunoglobulins. However, no hypersensitivity or other untoward reactions were observed in any of the patients studied, even when multiple repeat scans.

Monoclonal antibodies conjugated to ^{131}iodine, ^{123}iodine, and ^{111}indium are currently being studied by a number of investigators. Larsen and co-workers recently reported the results of imaging of 33 patients with advanced melanoma treated with ^{131}I-labeled Fab fragments specific for the p97 melanoma-associated antigen (35). Mach and co-workers have investigated ^{131}I-labeled anti-CEA monoclonal antibodies (36). Twenty-eight patients, 26 with large-bowel carcinomas and 2 with pancreatic carcinomas, were given injections of 0.3 mg ^{131}I-labeled anti-CEA, representing 1.0 to 1.5 mCi. In 14 of the 28 patients, a radioactive spot corresponding to the tumor was detected 36 to 48 hours after injection. In 6 patients, the scans were questionable, and in the remaining 8 patients, they were entirely negative. Epenetos and co-workers labeled monoclonal antibodies with ^{123}iodine and demonstrated that the ^{123}I-antibody conjugate detected antigens on ovarian, breast, and gastrointestinal neoplasms (37). They demonstrated specific localization and successful imaging in these patients. Similar results have been reported by other investigators (38,39).

In our own studies at the National Cancer Institute, antibody was coupled to diethylenetriaaminepentaacetic acid (DTPA) and was then labeled with ^{111}indium (^{111}In) just prior to infusion into patients with CTCL (Bunn et al., paper submitted). Patients were imaged with 1 mg of ^{111}In-DTPA-T101 mixed with either 10 or 50 mg of unlabeled T101. While there appeared to be considerable nonspecific activity in the bone marrow, liver, and spleen, excellent tumor localization was demonstrated. Tumor-involved lymph nodes as small as 0.5 cm that were not noted on physical examination and by standard diagnostic tests were identified with ^{111}In-DTPA-T101.

Therapeutic studies with radionuclides conjugated to antibodies are currently under way at a number of centers. Some of the pioneering work in this area has been reported by Order and co-workers (40). Radiolabeled ^{131}I anti-ferritin heterologous antiserum was used in treating hepatoma and anti-CEA in the treatment of biliary cancer. Doses of ^{131}I-labeled anti-ferritin as high as 150 mCi were given in single injections. A total of 24 hepatoma patients were treated, with 4 patients responding with partial responses. They have demonstrated that the hematologic toxicity is acceptable and that selected tumor targeting occurs despite the fact that there is ferritin in normal tissues and organs. They have shown that they can increase the half-life by diluting the high specific labeled ^{131}I anti-ferritin immunoglobulin with non-radíoactive anti-ferritin immunoglobulin. Therapeutic trials with monoclonal antibodies have been reported by Larsen and co-workers (35). Patients were treated with ^{131}I-labeled Fab fragments of an antibody directed to the p97 melanoma-associated antigen. Seven selected patients were treated with a cumulative dose of 130 to 529 mCi of ^{131}iodine. While objective tumor regression was not reported, those doses were very well tolerated, and excellent tumor localization was seen. Bone marrow toxicity appeared to be the dose-limiting toxicity for the ^{131}I-anti-p97.

We are currently preparing to carry out therapy trials for patients with CTCL and CLL using T101 conjugated to ^{125}I and ^{131}I. As these are radiosensitive tumors, they should be excellent targets for isotope therapy. Other anticipated immunoconjugate therapy trials for lymphoma patients will be drug and toxin conjugates using doxorubicin, vindesine, ricin, and gelonin conjugated to T101.

10. PURGING OF AUTOLOGOUS BONE MARROW WITH MONOCLONAL ANTIBODIES

Another attractive therapeutic application of monoclonal antibodies is to "clean up" autologous bone marrow prior to bone marrow transplantation. Patients with acute lymphoblastic leukemia have had bone marrow removed and treated with the J5 monoclonal antibody (41). Following bone marrow removal, treatment, and storage, patients were treated with high-dose chemotherapy and radiation therapy and then "rescued" with their J5 antibody-treated autologous bone marrow. A similar approach to therapy has been described using the B1 monoclonal antibody to clean up autologous bone marrow from patients with NHL (42). Eight patients with relapsed B-cell NHL were first induced into a minimum disease state (with less than 5% bone-marrow involvement with tumor). Bone marrow was then removed and treated with anti-B1 antibody and complement. Patients were then treated with intensive chemoradiotherapy and reconstituted with anti-B1 treated autologous bone marrow. All patients achieved a complete clinical response and engrafted by 8 weeks. There was no significant toxicity; B cells were detected by 2 months after transplantation and normal immunogloblin levels were achieved by 6 months. Six of 8 patients were disease free in unmaintained remission from 3 to 20 months after transplantation. The results of these trials are preliminary but have clearly demonstrated that antibody-treated autologous bone marrow is capable of restoring hematopoiesis. Long-term disease-free survival will be necessary before concluding that these therapies have been successful.

11. CONCLUSION

The use of monoclonal antibody and antibody immunoconjugates in the treatment and radioimaging of cancer is in its infancy. While much work needs to be done to clarify many of the issues surrounding the use of monoclonal antibodies, it has been clearly demonstrated in both animal tumor models and humans that antibody alone and antibody conjugates can be safely administered with minimal adverse effects and in selected cases have been shown to have diagnostic and therapeutic value. Problems such as nonspecific localization of antibody in the reticuloendothelial system, host antibody response, and antigenic heterogeneity are all major obstacles to safe and effective therapy with monoclonal antibodies. These issues are under investigation in animal models and humans. While anti-idiotype antibodies are highly specific and have demonstrated remarkable responses in a small number of patients, problems such as biclonality of some lymphomas, instability of the idiotype, and the difficulty in making "tailor-made" antibodies for individual patients clearly limit the role for anti-idiotype therapy. Purging of bone marrow with antibodies and complement (or coupled to toxins) is limited to only a few diseases. However, studies thus far have demonstrated that tumor cells can be removed from the bone marrow by in vitro treatment with antibody and complement, this treated bone marrow can successfully engraft, and a number of patients have been rendered disease free for over 1 year. This may prove to be an important application of monoclonal antibody therapy and it bypasses most of the problems with monoclonal antibody therapy described above. Perhaps the most important future role for monoclonal antibody therapy will be in patients with minimal disease in the "adjuvant" setting, where antibody conjugates may localize and destroy micrometastatic deposits of tumor cells. We remain cautiously optimistic in exploring these exciting new approaches to cancer therapy.

REFERENCES

1. Merigan TC, Sikora K, Breeden JH, Levy R, Rosenberg JA. 1978. Preliminary observations on the effect of human leukocyte interferon on non-Hodgkin's lymphoma. N Engl J Med 299:1449-1453.
2. Louie AC, Gallagher JG, Sikora K, Levy R, Rosenberg SA, Merigan TC. 1981. Follow-up observations on the effect of human leukocyte interferon on non-Hodgkin's lymphoma. Blood 58:712-718.
3. Gutterman J, Blumenschein G, Alexanian R, et al. 1980. Leukocyte interferon-induced tumor regression in human metastatic breast cancer, multiple myeloma, and malignant lymphoma. Ann Intern Med 93:399-406.
4. Sherwin SA, Knost JA, Fein S, et al. 1982. A multiple dose phase I trial of recombinant leukocyte A interferon in cancer patients. JAMA 248:2461-2466.
5. Quesada JR, Reuben J, Manning JR, Hersh EM, Gutterman JU. 1984. Alpha interferon for induction of remission in hairy-cell leukemia. N Engl J Med 310:15-18.
6. Foon KA, Sherwin SA, Abrams PG, et al. Recombinant leukocyte A interferon: An effective agent for the treatment of advanced non-Hodgkin's lymphoma. N Engl J Med, in press.
7. Foon KA, Bottino GC, Abrams PG, et al. Recombinant leukocyte A interferon is not an effective agent for the treatment of advanced chronic lymphocytic leukemia. Am J Med, in press.
8. Bunn PA, Foon KA, Ihde DC, et al. 1984. Recombinant leukocyte A interferon: An active agent in advanced cutaneous T cell lymphoma. Ann Intern Med 101:484-487.

9. The non-Hodgkin's lymphoma pathologic classification project. National Cancer Institute sponsored study of classification of non-Hodgkin's lymphoma. Summary and description of a working formulation for clinical usage. Cancer 49:2112-35, 1982.
10. Oldham RK. 1983. Monoclonal antibodies in cancer therapy. J Clin Oncol 1(9):582-590.
11. Levy R, Miller RA. 1983. Tumor therapy with monoclonal antibodies. Fed Proc 42:2650-2756.
12. Ritz J, Schlossman SF. 1982. Utilization of monoclonal antibodies in treatment of leukemia and lymphoma. Blood 59:1-11.
13. Ritz J, Pesando JM, Sallan SE, Clavell LA, Notis-McConarty J, Rosenthal P, Schlossman SF. 1981. Serotherapy of acute lymphoblastic leukemia with monoclonal antibody. Blood 58:141-152.
14. Nadler LM, Stashenko P, Hardy R, et al. 1980. Serotherapy of a patient with a monoclonal antibody directed against a human lymphoma-associated antigen. Cancer Res 40:3147-3154.
15. Dillman RO, Shawler DL, Sobel RE, et al. 1982. Murine monoclonal antibody therapy in two patients with chronic lymphocytic leukemia. Blood 59:1036-1045.
16. Dillman RO, Shawler DL, Dillman JB, Royston I. 1984. Therapy of chronic lymphocytic leukemia and cutaneous T-cell lymphoma with T101 monoclonal antibody. J Clin Oncol 2:881-891.
17. Foon KA, Schroff RW, Bunn PA, et al. 1984. Effects of monoclonal antibody therapy in patients with chronic lymphocytic leukemia. Blood, in press.
18. Miller RA, Maloney DG, McKillop J, Levy R. 1981. <u>In vivo</u> effects of murine hybridoma monoclonal antibody in a patient with T-cell leukemia. Blood 58:78-86.
19. Miller RA, Levy R. 1981. Response of cutaneous T cell lymphoma to therapy of hybridoma monoclonal antibody. Lancet 2:225-230.
20. Miller RA, Oseroff AR, Stratte PT, Levy R. 1983. Monoclonal antibody therapeutic trials in seven patients with T-cell lymphoma. Blood 62:988-995.
21. Foon KA, Schroff RW, Sherwin SA, Oldham RK, Bunn PA, Hsu S-M. 1983. Monoclonal antibody therapy of chronic lymphocytic leukemia and T cell lymphoma: Preliminary observations. In: Monoclonal Antibodies and Cancer. BD Boss, RE Langman, IS Towbridge, R Dulbecco, eds. Academic Press, New York, pp. 39-52.
22. Hatzubai A, Maloney DG, Levy R. 1981. Use of a monoclonal anti-idiotype antibody to study the biology of a human B cell lymphoma. J Immunol 126:2397-2402.
23. Miller RA, Maloney DG, Warnke R, Levy R. 1982. Treatment of B-cell lymphoma with monoclonal anti-idiotype antibody. N Engl J Med 306:517-522.
24. Lowder JN, Meeker TC, Maloney DG, Thielmans K, Miller RA, Levy R. 1984. Anti-idiotype monoclonal antibody therapy of human B lymphocytic malignancy. Proc Am Soc Clin Oncol 3:250.

25. Sklar J, Cleary ML, Thielemans K, Gralow J, Warnke R, Levy R. 1984. Biclonal B-cell lymphoma. N Engl J Med 311:20-27.
26. Raffeld M, Cossman J. 1984. Instability of idiotype in follicular lymphomas. Blood (Suppl. 1).
27. Oldham RK, Foon KA, Morgan AC, et al. 1984. Monoclonal antibody therapy of malignant melanoma: In vivo localization in cutaneous metastasis after intravenous administration. J Clin Oncol, in press.
28. Schroff RW, Farrell MM, Klein RA, Giardina SL, Oldham RK, Foon KA. 1984. T65 antigen modulation in a chronic lymphocytic leukemia phase I monoclonal antibody trial. J Immunol 133:1641-1648.
29. Schroff RW, Foon KA, Wilburn SB, Oldham RK, Morgan AC. 1984. Human anti-murine immunoglobulin responses in patients receiving monoclonal antibody therapy. Cancer Res, in press.
30. Sears HF, Herlyn D, Steplewski Z, Koprowski H. 1984. Effects of monoclonal antibody immunotherapy on patients with gastrointestinal adenocarcinoma. J Biol Resp Modif 3:138-150.
31. Foon KA, Bernhard MI, Oldham RK. 1982. Monoclonal antibody therapy: Assessment by animal tumor models. J Biol Resp Modif 1:277-304.
32. Goldenberg DM, DeLand FH. 1982. History and status of tumor imaging with radiolabeled antibodies. J Biol Resp Modif 1:121-136.
33. Goldenberg DM, DeLand FH, Kim EE, et al. 1978. Use of radiolabeled antibody to carcinoembryonic antigen for the detection and localization of diverse cancers by external photoscanning. N Engl J Med 298:1384-1388.
34. Mach J-P, Carrel S, Forni M, Ritschard J, Donath A, Alberto P. 1980. Tumor localization of radiolabeled antibodies against carcino-embryonic antigen in patients with carcinoma. N Engl J Med 303:5-10.
35. Larsen SM, Carresquillo JA, Krohn KA, et al. 1982. Localization of ^{131}I-labeled p97-specific Fab fragments in human melanoma as a basis for radiotherapy. J Clin Invest 72:2101-2114.
36. Mach J-P, Buchegger F, Forni M, et al. 1981. Use of radiolabeled monoclonal anti-CEA antibodies for detection of human carcinomas by external photoscanning and tomoscintigraphy. Immunol Today, December:239-249.
37. Epenetos AA, Britton KE, Mather S, et al. 1982. Targeting of mature 123-labeled tumour associated monoclonal antibodies to ovarian, breast, and gastrointestinal tumors. Lancet 2:999-1004.
38. Smedley HM, Finan P, Lennox ES, et al. 1983. Localization of metastatic carcinoma by a radiolabeled monoclonal antibody. Br J Cancer 47:253-259.
39. Fanands PA, Perkins AC, Pimm MV, et al. 1982. Radioimmunodetection of human colorectal cancers by an antitumour monoclonal antibody. Lancet 2:397-400.
40. Order SE, Klein JL, Leichner PK, Wharham MD, Ettinger DS, Siegelman SS. 1982. Advances in iodine 131-labeled antiferritin immunoglobulin cancer therapy. Cancer Bulletin 34: 264-267.

41. Ritz J, Bast RC, Clavell LA, et al. 1982. Autologous bone marrow transplantation in CALLA-positive acute lymphoblastic leukemia after in vitro treatment with J5 monoclonal antibody and complement. Lancet 2:60-63.
42. Nadler L, Takvorian T, Botnick L, et al. 1984. Anti-B1 monoclonal antibody and complement treatment in autologous bone-marrow transplantation for relapsed B-cell non-Hodgkin's lymphoma. Lancet 2:427-431.

A COMPARISON OF THE ACQUIRED IMMUNE DEFICIENCY SYNDROME IN MONKEY AND MAN

PAUL R. MEYER, KENT G. OSBORN*

SUMMARY

Spontaneous acquired immunodeficiencies occurring among selected humans and in primate colonies throughout the United States have a number of clinical, pathologic, immunologic, and biologic similarities.[1,2] These include a relatively restricted geographic pattern[3,4] and opportunistic infections and tumors;[5-8] more recently a retrovirus is proposed as the causative factor in both.[9,10] This chapter outlines common features and details a pathomechanistic approach to the understanding of the disease syndrome(s).

AIDS IN THE HUMAN

Based on the definition and complications outlined in Table 1, Centers for Disease Control (CDC)[11] has sought and received over 8,000 (1984) reports of life threatening opportunistic infection, Kaposi's sarcoma and primary central nervous system lymphoma as part of its epidemiologic investigation of the acquired immune deficiency syndrome.[12] Prior to this outbreak, such serious complications were seen primarily in the intentionally immunosuppressed or secondarily immunocompromised host. The age population has been in general healthy prior to the onset of the syndrome, with the majority of the patients (85%) being between the ages of 20 and 50 years. Over 90% of the patients belong to four high-risk groups: homosexual males (75%),[13,14] intravenous (IV) drug abusers with no history of homosexual behavior (13%),[15,16] factor VIII deficient males (0.3%),[17,18] or Haitian immigrants (6%).[19] The remaining cases (5%) have been grouped into the category "no risk factors." This category includes heterosexual women (sexual

*Kent G. Osborn, DVM, California Regional Primate Center, University of California at Davis, Davis, California.

Table 1. Case Definition--Acquired Immune Deficiency Syndrome (AIDS)*

1. Presence of a reliably diagnosed disease at least moderately indicative of underlying cellular immunodeficiency (eg, Kaposi's sarcoma in a patient <60 years of age, *Pneumocystis carinii* pneumonia).

2. Absence of known causes of underlying immunodeficiency and of any other reduced resistance reported to be associated with the disease (eg, immunosuppressive therapy, lymphoreticular malignancy).

DISEASES FULFILLING THE CENTERS FOR DISEASE CONTROL DEFINITION: (The following disorders appear disseminated and persistent)

A. Protozoan Infections

Pneumocystis carinii
Toxoplasma gondii
Cryptospiridium

B. Fungal Infections

Candida
Cryptococcus

C. Bacteria

Mycobacterium avium-intracellulare

D. Viral Infections

Herpes Simplex
Cytomegalovirus
Progressive Multifocal leukoencephalopathy

E. Cancers

Kaposi's sarcoma
Non-Hodgkin lymphoma

*Case definition as defined by Centers for Disease Control (CDC), Atlanta, Georgia, to be used for "epidemiologic" surveillance.

partners of bisexual men or hemophilic men),[15] transfusion recipients,[20] prison inmates,[21] and children of patients in high risk groups.[16,19]

The largest number of patients are male (95%) and white (58%), although blacks (25%), hispanics (14%), and Haitians (6%) may have an incidence higher than their proportion in the total U.S. population.[11,12] Remarkedly, no case of AIDS has been reported in an Asian.

Most reports originate from four major U.S. metropolitan areas: New York City, New York (38%), Newark, New Jersey (30%), San Francisco, California (12%), Los Angeles, California (8%) and Miami, Florida (4%). The disease has a doubling time of six to eight months. While only 593 reports were received between June 1, 1981 and September 16, 1982, over 2300 cases have been described between January and December of 1983. An additional 4000 cases were described in 1984. The disease is spreading, with additional cases now being described in Central and South America, Africa, Europe and Australia.[22,23]

The cumulative case fatality rate exceeds 60% for cases diagnosed more than one year ago and up to 100% for those cases diagnosed more than three years ago. No case report has been published documenting full immunologic recovery of a patient with AIDS, so that the case fatality may approach 100%.

The disease is apparently transmissible and a number of case studies have described the interlinking sexual partnerships between AIDS patients.[24] Not surprisingly, the complicating tumors and infections appear interrelated with Kaposi's sarcoma, *Pneumocystis carinii* pneumonia, and other opportunistic infections being described in common sexual partners. More recently, study of transfusion patients has shown that a predictable incubation period exists. In 62 adults who received from 1 to 60 units of blood (mean 14.3), the median incubation time from transfusion to onset of AIDS was 28 months (range 5-62 months). In this same study, an analysis of 12 children showed a somewhat shorter period, with a mean of 19.4 months (range 4-46 months). Children received a somewhat smaller quantity of blood (mean 15.6).[20]

Thus from the epidemiologic data, the acquired immune deficiency syndrome seems to have all the hallmarks of an infectious transmissible disease: common sexual partners, restriction to certain "risk" groups, geographic clustering and a predictable incubation time.

Recently the question of genetic susceptibility has been raised, based upon studies of the HLA system. Studies from New York have found that those patient displaying epidemic Kaposi's sarcoma (AIDS) as well as those having endemic Kaposi's sarcoma (non-AIDS) have an increased incidence of HLA-Dr5 and a suggestion of decreased incidence of HLA-Dr2. This findings have also been described in the polyadenopathy or pre-AIDS syndrome.[25]

Figure 1 shows the curve of AIDS cases for San Francisco, New York, and Los Angeles. Based on such studies, one can calculate the number of cases of AIDS in San Francisco and Los Angeles over the next two years.

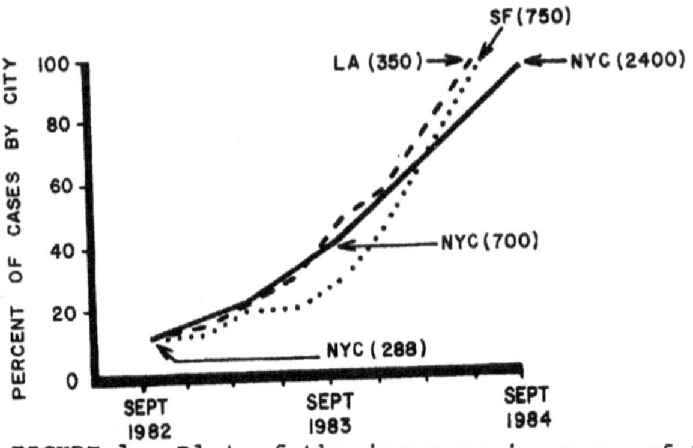

FIGURE 1. Plot of the increase in cases of AIDS in New York, San Francisco, and Los Angeles. Numbers are represented as 100% allowing one to predict that San Frnacisco will see another 1800 cases in the next year and Los Angeles another 2000 cases in the next two years. Data from "AIDS Task Force--New York, San Francisco, and Los Angeles."

AIDS IN THE SIMIAN (SAIDS)

An epizootic of acquired immunodeficiency has been identified in Rhesus-Macaques (Macca mulatta) at the California Regional Primate Center, University of California at Davis (UCD), and in other primate research centers throughout the United States.[4,26,27] At UCD, the epizootic involves a group of juvenile and young adult animals housed in a half-acre outdoor corral (NC-1). Retrospectively the outbreak was first noted in 1969.[28] Since that time, there has been at least three other outbreaks with an unusually high mortality rate (27.5% versus 5.5% in other unaffected cages). These past three outbreaks as well as recent transmittable cases have been defined on the basis of the criteria outlined in Table 2.[10] A comparison of human (Table 1) and monkey (Table 2) shows many similarities in the complicating infections and tumors that define AIDS and SAIDS.

Despite the relatively long period (15 years), episodic nature, and complex array of diseases in the simian immunodeficiency, the remaining nine half acre corrals have remained free from the SAIDS defined disorders. In fact, the periodicity and episodic nature of the syndrome may in large part be due to an attempt to conserve the remaining animals by introduction of new, young female animals into the corral. It should be noted that the higher incidence of female SAIDS is in large part due to inability to

Table 2. Case Definition--Simian Acquired Immune Deficiency Syndrome (SAIDS)*

Generalized lymphadenopathy must be present as well as at least four of the following findings

Splenomegaly	Bone marrow hyperplasia
Neutropenia (<1700)	Persistent diarrhea
Lymphopenia (<1600)	Mucocutaneous infection
Weight loss (>10%)	Opportunistic infection
Anemia (PCV < 30%)	Tumors: lymphoma, KS-like
Abnormal peripheral blood monocytes	

SAIDS ASSOCIATED INFECTIONS:

A. Protozoan

E. histolytica
E. coli
Cryptospiridium
Giardia
Trichimonas
Toxoplasmosis
Hexamita

B. Fungal

C. albicans

C. Bacteria

Campylobacter
Shigella
Klebsiella
Yersinia
S. aureus
S. pneumonia

D. Viral

CMV
Herpes simiae
SV 40
Paramyxovirus

*Case definition as proposed by California Regional Primate Center (UCD).

introduce larger number of competitive breeding males into the corral. Such an introduction would result in a genocide of the newer males by the older breeding males. Moreover, the issue of homosexuality in the monkey is more apparent than real. The hierarchical system of a mature breeding colony requires the submission of animals enforced by biting and scratching. Observers agree that there is not actual penetration or ejaculation in male-to-male encounters.

Recently the SAIDS syndrome was shown to be transmissible monkey-to-monkey using SAIDS plasma, blood, saliva and lymph node products.[2,6,29-31] The incubation time from inoculation to death varied from one to nine months and the clinical course included a prodrome of neutropenia, adenopathy, splenomegaly and diarrhea. At post-mortem examination, these animals were found to have diseases fulfilling the SAIDS case definition (Table 2).

PATHOGENESIS (Lymph Node Findings in Monkey and Man)

The fully developed diseases in the monkey and in the human share a number of common opportunistic infections and unusual tumors (Tables 1 and 2). Moreover, the prodrome compromises a number of similar immunologic syndromes (Table 3).[10,32] In an attempt to investigate the pathogenesis, we undertook a comparison of lymph node biopsies obtained in spontaneous human cases with those from experimentally inoculated animals and compared our findings to those of reactive normal controls in both primates.[33,34]

The majority of human lymph node biopsy specimens came from patients on a protocol study at the Norris Cancer Center/LAC-USC Medical Center. These patients had the syndrome of persistent generalized lymphadenopathy (PGL) (Table 3). PGL has been linked epidemiologically and clinically with the acquired immunodeficiency syndrome. The syndrome has been described in most "risk group" members and includes homosexual men,[31] hemophiliac children,[18]

Table 3. Prodromal Signs and Symptoms of (S)AIDS

AIDS Related Complex (ARC)*

The case definition for AIDS may not include the full spectrum of manifestations, which may range from absence of symptoms (despite laboratory evidence of immune deficiency) to nonspecific symptoms (e.g., fever, weight loss, generalized persistent lymphadenopathy, neutropenia) to specific diseases that are insufficiently predictive of cellular immunodeficiency to be included in incidence monitoring (e.g., tuberculosis, oral candidiasis, herpes zoster) to malignant neoplasms that cause as well as result from immunodeficiency. Some of the clinical disorders commonly found in patients with ARC include cutaneous and oral fungal infections, chronic diarrhea, persistent generalized lymphadenopathy, idiopathic thrombocytopenic purpura, nephrotic syndrome, and in younger primates failure to thrive with chronic and persistent infections. Often, further testing of the immune system is necessary before "other conventional or drug-induced" causes of these disorders can be ruled out.

Case Definition--Persistent Generalized Lymphadenopathy (PGL)*

PGL is defined as lymphadenopathy of unexplained cause in two or more extrainguinal sites for at least three months duration. If a biopsy is undertaken, the histology is that of a reactive follicular hyperplasia.

---

*These definitions are general guidelines applied to human and are NOT rigid criteria. They may also be generally useful for the monkey (eg, lymphadenopathy is a common initial finding in inoculated monkeys and may occur throughout the course).

Haitians,[19] female sexual partners of male hemophiliacs[35] and transfusion recipients.[20] In one study from our institution, we found it impossible to separate on clinical findings alone those men who had acquired immune deficiency syndrome from those men with only the reactive polyadenopathy syndrome. Therefore, it has been our practice to biopsy all such men at the time of presentation.[36]

In the monkey inoculated with plasma, blood, lymph node homogenates and saliva, the disease has been transmitted. As noted above, before opportunistic infections occur (SAIDS), features of the AIDS-related complex, including polyadenopathy and hepatosplenomegaly, may appear from one to six weeks after inoculation.[29,34] These animals have been biopsied periodically every three months; however, if the disease appears to be progressing and/or other clinical reasons become evident, a biopsy is taken more often.

Two patterns of lymph node reaction have been defined in both monkey and man. Exuberant follicular hyperplasia is the most common reaction, although lymphoid depletion is also seen.[37] Davis et al found in a study of 66 men (56 follicular hyperplasia and 10 follicular involution--lymphoid depletion) that only one patient in the follicular group developed a malignancy, while malignancies were noted in four of the follicular involution group ($P<0.001$).[38] Lymphoid depletion is the most common finding in both monkey and man at necropsy/autopsy. In addition to the clinical similarities and lymph node morphology (Figures 2 and 3) there was a comparable distribution of cells having T, B, and monocyte phenotype. Figure 2 and 3 outline the morphologic similarities; Figure 4, the phenotypic findings.[18,33,39]

Control lymph node specimens in monkey and man differed qualitatively and quantitatively from the reactive follicular hyperplasia seen in PGL patients and in inoculated SAIDS animals. Reactive follicles in controls were well organized and round ($B-1^+$) with small well-defined mantle zones (IgD^+) near the medullary aspect of the lymph node. The majority of follicle associated T cells were of helper phenotype ($OKT-4^+$, $Leu-3^+$), while few cells were of suppressor type ($Leu-2^+$, $Leu-2A^+$, Cappel suppressor/ cytotoxic T^+) were present. The ratio of helper: suppressor phenotype was between 2:1 to 3:1. Monocyte macrophage phenotype ($OKM-1^+$) were inconsistently present within the follicular centers. Dendritic cells ($CM-1^+$) presented a uniform cohesive pattern within

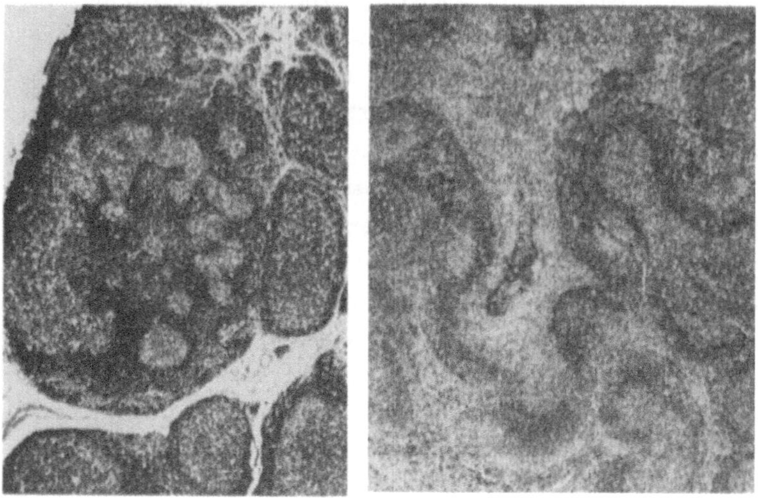

FIGURE 2. Section of lymph node: monkey (left) and man (right). The histologic pattern of the node is dominated by an exuberant follicular hyperplasia.

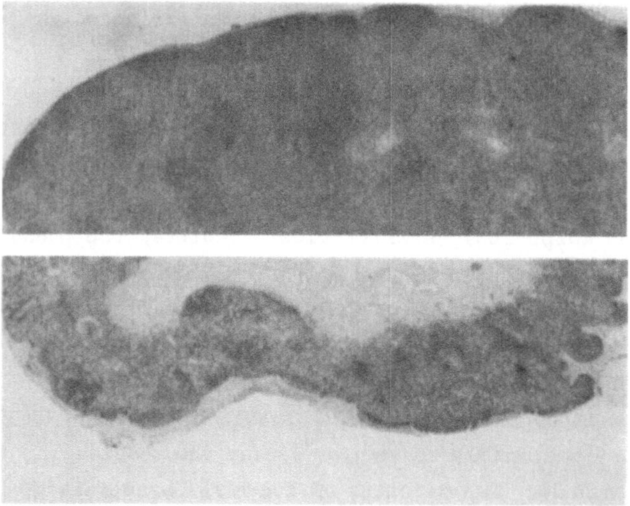

FIGURE 3. Section of lymph node: monkey (upper) and man (lower). The lymph node appears atrophic with no remaining follicular centers and few small lymphocyte areas (dark).

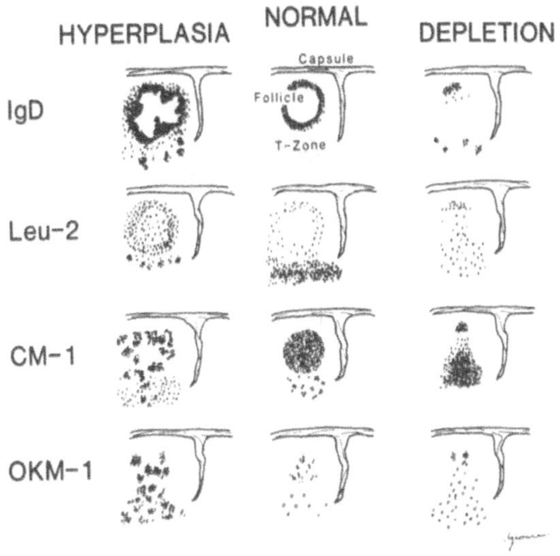

FIGURE 4. Summary of immunostaining results. A comparison of selected antibodies in control lymph nodes with reactions in (S)AIDS-complex.

The atypical follicular hyperplasia of (S)AIDS shows large misshaped mantle (IgD) with an increase in T suppressor/cytotoxic phenotype (Leu-2) in the central follicle. The follicular reticulum cell (CM-1) staining is diminished and no longer cohesive. Increasing numbers of mature monocytes/macrophages (OKM-1) start in follicle and paracortex.

In the lymphoid depletion stage the follicular disruption is far advanced with loss of demarcation between mantle cells (IgD) and areas of B-cell transformation. Dendritic cell staining (CM-1) is isolated to occasional small islands or completely absent. Increases in monocyte/macrophages (CM-1, OKM-1) become more prominent within residual B- and T-cell areas as other cell types begin to disappear.

Summary of antibody specificity:

- IgD - Immunoglobulin D heavy chain
- Leu-2 - Suppressor/cytotoxic T cell
- CM-1 - Dendritic follicular center cell antibody; some monocyte cross-reactivity
- OKM-1 - Mature peripheral blood monocyte and mature macrophage

the follicles with a distinctive smooth border separating mantle areas from areas of transformation. In T-dependent paracortical regions, cells bearing helper and suppressor phenotypes were uniformly present in large numbers. Occasional OKM-1^+ and CM-1^+ cells were present. The anatomic locations of positive cells corresponds to published reports in man and monkey.[18,33,39]

The designation of a lymphocyte depletion or follicular hyperplasia was based on the number and appearance of geographic areas containing large transformed B cells or morphologically typical follicular centers (Figures 2 and 3). While occasional lymphocyte depleted nodes (Figure 3) contained follicular centers, none contain more than three per section, and such remaining follicles were often poorly formed.

Early Changes in SAIDS (Monkey)

The earliest post-inoculation change (10 days to three weeks) in the monkey was an expansion of the interfollicular region from a proliferation of transformed immunoblastic T cells (Leu-$2A^+$ or OKT-4^+), with or without an associated follicular hyperplasia. Cortical blastic expansion evolved into either lymphocyte depletion in 5-12 weeks or to follicular hyperplasia in 5-36 weeks. As the time between biopsies varied, the precise interval could not be determined. This blastic reaction was only rarely seen in humans.[37]

Follicular Hyperplasia

An exuberant atypical follicular hyperplasia was present in homosexual man and inoculated monkeys. This reaction was characterized by large, ill-formed and irregularly shaped, follicular centers (Figure 2), well emphasized by B-1 and IgD staining and differing from that seen in controls. IgD^+ cells were no longer confined to the immediate perifollicular area and were often present in the areas of B cell transformation and/or dispersed into the surrounding T cell areas. These suppressor/cytotoxic cells (by phenotype) often predominated over helper/inducer phenotype within the follicular centers in the mantle. The helper/suppressor ratio was 1 or less. Dendritic cells (CM-1^+) showed a patchy staining and/or diminution in numbers. In paracortical T cell areas, the absolute numbers of helper and suppressor cells were variably decreased. Helper T cells predominated over suppressor cells within the T-dependent paracortical areas. Macrophage/monocyte (OKM-1^+, CM-1^+) varied in predominence, generally paralleling the increase in the suppressor/cytotoxic T cells within the follicular center.

In an early study, eight monkeys inoculated with SAIDS material died of SAIDS. At the time of death, two of the lymph nodes showed pronounced follicular hyperplasia. Both animals had a prolonged disease course after inoculation, dying at seven and nine months with multiple disease features fulfilling the SAIDS definition (Table 2). While living, all eight inoculated monkeys had biopsy specimens characterized by abnormal follicular hyperplasia. These animals have had some of the prodromal signs and symptoms of SAIDS (Table 3). By comparison, follicular hyperplasia is the most often recognized pattern by morphology in human biopsy material from patients at risk for AIDS. Two of the five homosexual men in our study had Kaposi's sarcoma in the same lymph node, thereby fulfilling the CDC criteria for AIDS (Table 1, Figure 2).[12]

Lymphocyte Depletion

The lymphocyte depleted lymph node showed profound alteration in morphology and immunostaining (Figures 3 and 4). Few clear cut areas of B cell activation (follicular centers) were present. Frequently, the only method of identifying such a residual small B cell area was by immunostaining (B-1^+, IgD^+). These antibodies fail to draw a distinction between areas of mantle and transformed cells. Serial sections were performed to determine the comparative distribution of phenotypes. Total cells bearing T helper/inducer (Leu-3^+, OKT-4^+) and T suppressor/cytotoxic phenotype (Leu-2^+, Leu-$2A^+$, Cappel suppressor/cytotoxic T^+) were reduced, especially within T dependent paracortical areas. Dendritic cell staining (CM-1^+) was absent or severely reduced. Macrophages (OKM-1^+, CM-1^+) were increased in all areas of the lymph node. Six of the eight animals dying of SAIDS showed the lymphocyte depletion pattern at postmortem examination. In contrast to the two animals dying with follicular hyperplasia, these animals had a rapid course, dying 5-12 weeks post-inoculation. The cause of death included a variety of opportunistic infectious agents which fulfill the SAIDS case definition (Table 2). With the exception of only one of our human patients, all with a lymphocyte depletion morphologic pattern fulfill the CDC case definition for AIDS, having Kaposi's sarcoma or Pneumocystis carinii pneumonia. By morphology lymphocyte depletion is the most frequent finding at autopsy/necropsy in men and monkeys dying from AIDS/SAIDS.[5,7]

Summary Of Lymph Node Findings

Lymph nodes from infected monkeys and AIDS-infected humans show a similar morphologic profile as well as qualitative and quantitative microanatomic changes in mononuclear cell subsets (Figures 2, 3 and 4). The follicular centers become poorly formed and distorted as the disease progresses. Cellular organization within B cell areas and the reticulum cell network are disrupted. Distribution, ratios and absolute numbers of subsets are altered. There is an increase of the suppressor cell phenotype within the follicular center. In humans, the helper phenotype is more depleted than the suppressor phenotype in both lymph nodes and peripheral blood, while in the monkey, this occurred less consistently. Ultimately, in the lymphocyte depletion stage, marked disruption of the B cell area occurs accompanied by infiltration of macrophages.

In Figure 5, an attempt is made to define the alteration seen within the lymph node follicle using the Lukes-Collins follicular center cell concept. The AIDS agent infects B cells causing a profound stimulus to the B-cell arm of the immune system. Antibodies are produced in an attempt to suppress this agent; however, the limited extracellular range of a retrovirus makes this antibody response ineffective. The suppressor cells attempt to suppress this pronounced follicular response. If this succeeds, then immunosuppression may intervene. If this fails, then a B cell lymphoma may result. Thus it seems that in the lymph node, at least, the primary stimulus is to the B-cell arm with three possible consequences: (1) development of B cell lymphomas, (2) development of profound immuno-failure with the complications of opportunistic infections, and (3) continued immunologic warfare with persistence of the syndrome. In the human this evolution from persistent generalized lymphadenopathy syndrome to AIDS or lymphoma may vary from 3%-6% per year, while in the inoculated monkey such a progression occurs in well over 50% per year. The factors determining disease and the progression between follicular and

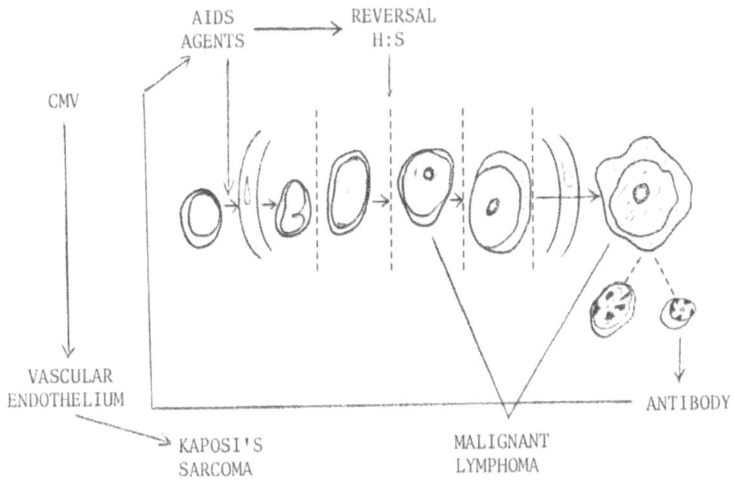

FIGURE 5. Schema outlining the development of AIDS, PGL, and lymphoma using the follicular center cell concept of Lukes/Collins. The AIDS agent(s) may infect B lymphocytes leading to an increase in T-suppressor cells in an attempt to diminish this B-cell proliferation. If such a response is successful or the AIDS agent(s) infects other cells, then immune failure intervenes and the patient dies of complicating infections and tumors. If the suppression fails then clonal B-cell evolution occurs and the patient develops a monoclonal B-cell lymphoma. More commonly, this immunologic warfare continues with immune function altered. The antibodies produced by this B-cell proliferation are ineffective due to the limited extracellular range of the retrovirus.

lymphocyte depletion patterns are complex and involve the interaction of normal immune mechanisms, factors contributed by infectious agent, genetic and environmental factors, as well as therapy.

MALIGNANT LYMPHOMA OF B-CELL ORIGIN

Non-Hodgkin's lymphomas occurring in the background of acquired immune deficiency have been reported from New York City, Houston, San Francisco, Miami, and Los Angeles.[40] Cancer registry data from the San Francisco Bay area as well as Los Angeles County have indicated up to a three-fold rise in lymphomas in the young, never married men over the same time period (Table 4). Recent reports from the New England Regional Primate Center have demonstrated the transmissibility of malignant B cell-derived lymphomas (Burkitt and B-immunoblastic sarcoma types) in the monkey.[6] We,

Table 4. Incidence of Burkitt's Lymphoma Agmong All Non-Hodgkin Lymphoma (Los Angeles County, California)*

	MARRIED	
	Male	Female
1978-82	1.0%	1.0%
	SINGLE	
	Male	Female
1978-80	1.0%	1.0%
1981-82	16.0%	1.0%

*Cancer Surveillance Program--Los Angeles County California.

too, have seen the evolution of a Burkitt-type lymphoma in a monogamous homosexual pair.[41]

In a collaborative multicenter study with Ziegler et al,[40] the findings in 90 homosexual men with malignant lymphoma were reported. The median age was 37 years, and the age distribution was identical to that seen for the AIDS cases reported to the CDC. Sixty-two percent were of high grade, 29% of intermediate grade, and 7% low grade. Histologic subtypes and malignant-cell phenotypes were those of B-cell origin. Eighty-eight of the 90 men presented with extranodal lymphoma. Central nervous system, bone marrow, gut and mucocutaneous sites were the most frequent. Mortality and morbidity showed a close relationship to the prodromal manifestations: 29 men presented with AIDS and 19 are dead or ill (91%); 33 men presented with generalized lymphadenopathy and 26 are dead or ill (79%); 12 have no prodromal manifestations and five (42%) are dead or ill. Overall survival rates, analyzed according to histologic grade, were inferior to current survival rates in other patient populations. Relapses were common. Primary lymphoma of the brain confirmed a poor prognosis and only two of eleven patients diagnosed antimortem are alive today. Observations of a natural history disclosed progression to the disorders diagnostic of AIDS in 14 of 33 men who presented with generalized lymphadenopathy and in three of 12 without prodromes. Of 33 lymphomas examined, 30 were reported to display surface monoclonal immunoglobulins. Three lymphomas lacked surface immunoglobulins which stain positively with monoclonal reagents against B cells.

In a more detailed study from the Los Angeles County-USC Medical Center,[42] we found that the epidemic form of malignant lymphoma can be distinguishable from the endemic or background cases using the criteria outlined in Table 5. As in the monkey model, the majority of our human patients had either a Burkitt or B cell-derived immunoblastic sarcoma (Figure 6). Moreover, the observation of monoclonal "reactive" lymph nodes in homosexual men may suggest that the PGL syndrome is a prelymphomatous state.[37]

THE RETROVIRUS (Comparison of HTLV-III and the SAID Retrovirus)

Recent studies in both human and monkey have linked the transmission of AIDS/SAIDS to an RNA retrovirus. A brief summary of the findings and implications in the transmission of this agent will be outlined.

The AIDS and SAIDS retroviruses seem comparable in their RNA core, their magnesium dependent reverse transcriptase, and their ability to infect cells of the T cell lineage as well as B cells, particularly those previously infected by Epstein-Barr virus (EBV). In tissue culture, both agents appear to form characteristic syncytia.[9,10,29] At the electron microscopic level, the pictures provided by Gallo[9] and Marks[29] show an enveloped virus with a bullet-shaped core. Immunologic studies suggest that the human T

Table 5. Non-Hodgkin Lymphoma of Aggressive B-Cell Type: Features of Endemic and Epidemic Lymphoma.*

	ENDEMIC	EPIDEMIC
AGE	child, older adult	middle age (m=36)
SEX	m:f = 1:2	M:F = 1:0
SITE	node:extra-nodal 50:50	nodal:extra-nodal 3:24
EBV+	less than 30%	100%
HTLV+	less than 10%	greater than 90%
H/S r	greater than 1.0	less than 1.0 in 80%
HISTORY	autoimmune disease	multiple infections drug abuse

EBV=Epstein-Barr virus
HTLV=Human T-cell leukemia virus (III)
H/S r=Helper/suppressor ratio reversal

*Data taken from reference 42.

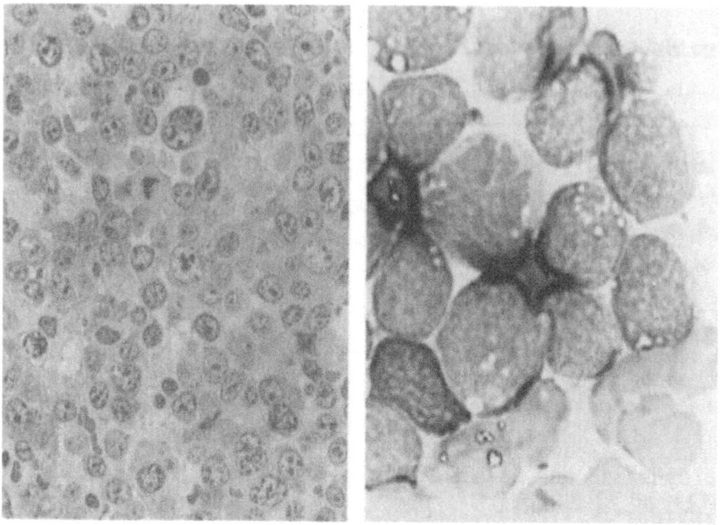

FIGURE 6. Malignant lymphoma of B-cell type: human--Burkitt's lymphoma (left) and B-immunoblastic sarcoma (right). Both monkey and man have developed Burkitt's lymphoma and immunoblastic sarcoma as a complication of HTLV-III infection. These lymphomas apparently occur in the setting of AIDS and persistent generalized lymphadenopathy (PGL), as well as in those without prodrome.

cell leukemia virus (HTLV-III) is a type C particle, while the monkey SAIDS retrovirus is characterized as a type D. Recently, in a comparative study, the two human retroviruses, lymphadenopathic associated virus (LAV) and HTLV-III, appeared to be identical agents.

In many ways, the (S)AIDS retroviruses appear to cause a disease in both monkey and man which parallels the course of hepatitis B (Table 6). The majority of patients who confront the agent (Table 6--left) apparently have an asymptomatic course and can only be identified by antibody studies and/or reversal of the helper/suppressor cell ratios. This, of course, corresponds to the anicteric, asymptomatic course of hepatitis B, diagnosable only by laboratory test for liver injury or convalescent antibodies to HbAg. The long-term effects of this exposure to (S)AIDS agents are presently unknown, although most patients have a stable course in the short term. Another group confronting the (S)AIDS agents (Table 6--right) reacts adversely to the virus by demonstrating a profound immune failure with a lymphocyte depletion pattern on lymph node morphology. The counterpart to hepatitis B is the rare

Table 6. Course Following Infection with (S)AIDS Agent(s), paralleling course of hepatitis B.

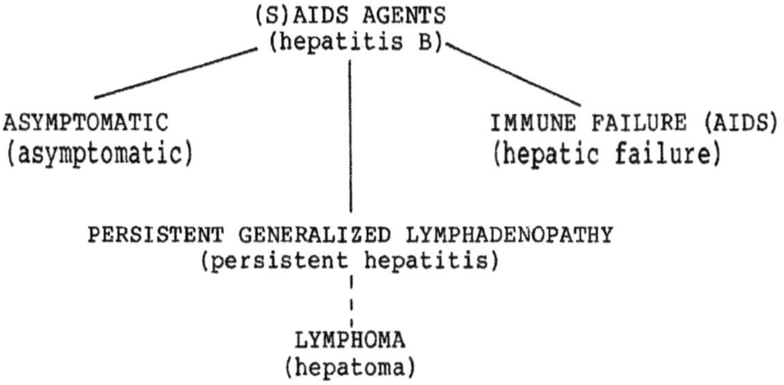

individual who develops fulminant hepatic failure. Finally, a third group (Table 6--center) follows a more prolonged but symptomatic course with polyadenopathy syndrome from which HTLV-III can be cultured. This "carrier" state is analogous to persistent or chronic active hepatitis in which hepatitis B antigen can be found. The outcome of this (S)AIDS carrier state is presently unknown, although progression to opportunistic tumors and infections occurs in a variable number of patients.

TRANSMISSION OF AIDS

Recent studies in both monkey and man has determined that the retrovirus associated with SAIDS is found not only in blood, plasma and lymph node, but that the agent may be cultured and demonstrated in saliva and semen.[43-46] It has been generally acknowledged that within the monkey, the behavioral patterns, including cleaning and grooming as well as hierarchical dominance enforcements by biting and scratching, may be a preferred mode of transmission. Recently in a retrospective study, an asymptomatic carrier from the California Regional Primate Center (UCD) was identified. This animal was housed in the corral NC-I and apparently spread the disorder to 34 other monkeys over a prolonged three year period. This spread included two of her own offspring.[43] More recently, an asymptomatic carrier state has been proposed within the human.[44-46] Here too, a mother apprently transmitted the disease to two children. Studies in both human and monkey show that those individuals with infected saliva make up about 40%-50% of the group from which virus can be cultured from peripheral blood lymphocyes. This may have profound implications for the transmission of the disease. We have recently seen two men with AIDS who frequented prostitutes and had no other risk factors. Thus, it seems likely that saliva and other body secretions may be involved in the clinical transmission of AIDS in the human as well as the monkey.

ADDENDUM

Recently, plasma contaminated with human retrovirus (HTLV-III) has been used to transmit the polyadenopathy syndrome to chimpanzees.[47]

REFERENCES

1. Fauci AS, Macher AM, Longo DL, et al. 1984. Acquired immunodeficiency syndrome: Epidemiologic, clinical, immunologic and therapeutic considerations. Ann Intern Med 100:92.
2. Gravell M, London WT, Houff SA, et al. 1984. Transmission of simian acquired immunodeficiency syndrome (SAIDS) with blood or filtered plasma. Science 223:74.
3. Centers for Disease Control. 1983. Update: Acquired immunodeficiency syndrome (AIDS)--United States. MMWR 32:465-467.
4. Hendrickson RV, Maul DH, Lerche NW, et al. 1984. Clinical features of acquired immunodeficiency in rhesus monkeys. Lab Ann Sci 34:140-145.
5. Osborn KG, Prahalada S, Lowenstine LJ, et al. 1984. The pathology of an epizootic of acquired immunodeficiency in rhesus macaques. Am J Pathol 114:94.
6. Hunt RD, Black BJ, Chalifoux LV, et al. 1983. Transmission of naturally occurring lymphoma in macaque monkeys. Proc Natl Acad Sci USA 80:5085.
7. Hui AN, Koss MN, Meyer PR. 1984. Necropsy findings in acquired immunodeficiency syndrome: A comparison of premortem diagnoses with postmortem findings. Hum Pathol 15:670.
8. Levine AM, Meyer PR, Begandy MK, et al. 1984. Development of B-cell lymphoma in homosexual men. Ann Intern Med 100:7.
9. Gallo RC, Salahuddin SZ, Popovic M, Shearer GM, Kaplan M, Haynes BF, Palker TJ, Redfield R, Oleski J, Safai B, White G, Foster P, Markham PD. 1984. Frequent detection and isolation of cytopathic retroviruses (HTLV-III) from patients with AIDS and at risk for AIDS. Science 224:500-503.
10. Gardner M, Marx P, Maul D, Osborn K, Hendrickson R, Lerche N, Munn B, Brunken B, Bryant M. 1984. Simian AIDS--Evidence for a retroviral etiology. Hematol Oncol 2:259-268.
11. Centers for Disease Control. 1982. Update on Kaposi's sarcoma and opportunistic infections in previously healthy persons--United States. MMWR 31:294.
12. Selik RM, Haverkos HW, Curran JW. 1984. Acquired immune deficiency syndrome (AIDS) trends in the United States, 1978-1982. Am J Med 76:493-500.
13. Gottlieb MS, Schroff R, Schanker HM, Weismann JD, Fan PT, Wolf RN, Saxon A. 1981. Pneumocystic carinii pneumonia and mucosal candidiasis in previously healthy homosexual men. N Engl J Med 305:1425-1431.

14. Masur H, Michelis MA, Greene JB, et al. 1981. An outbreak of community-acquired *Pneumocystic carinii* pneumonia: initial manifestation of cellular immune dysfunction. N Engl J Med 305:1431-1438.
15. Masur H, Michelis MA, Wormser GP, et al. 1982. Opportunistic infection in previously healthy women. Ann Intern Med 97:533-539.
16. Rubinstein A, Sicklick M, Gupta A, et al. 1983. Acquired immunodeficiency with reversed T4/T8 ratios in infants born to promiscuous and drug-addicted mother. J Am Med Assoc 249:2350-2356.
17. Luban NLC, Kelleher Jr JF, Reamon GH. 1983. Altered distribution of T-lymphocyte subpopulations in children and adolescents with hemophilia. Lancet 1:503-505.
18. Meyer PR, Modlin RL, Powars D, Ewing N, Parker JW, Taylor CR. 1983. Altered distribution of T-lymphocyte subpopulations in lymph nodes from patients with acquired immunodeficiency-like syndrome and hemophilia. J Pediatr 103:407-410.
19. Joneas JH, DeLage G, Chad Z, Lapointe N. 1983. Acquired immunodeficiency in infants born of Haitian mothers. N Engl J Med 308:842.
20. Curran JW, Lawrence DN, Jaffe H, et al. 1984. Acquired immunodeficiency syndrome (AIDS) associated with transfusions. N Engl J Med 310:69-75.
21. Wormser GP, Krupp LB, Hanrahan JP, et al. 1983. Acquired immunodeficiency syndrome in male prisoners. New insights into an emerging syndrome. Ann Int Med 98:297-303.
22. Glauser MP, Francioli P. 1984. Clinical and epidemiological survey of acquired immunodeficiency syndrome in Europe. Eur J Clin Microbiol 3:55-58.
23. Chumeck N, Mascart-Lemone F, DeMaubeuge J, Renez D, Marcelis L. 1983. Acquired immune deficiency syndrome in black Africans. Lancet 1:642.
24. Auerbach DM, Darrow WM, Jaffe HW, et al. 1984. Cluster of cases of acquired immune deficiency syndrome: patient's linked by sexual contact. Am J Med 76:487-492.
25. Metroka CE. 1984. Generalized lymphadenopathy in homosexual men: the epidemic of Kaposi's sarcoma and opportunistic infections. In: AIDS, Friedman-Kien AE, Laubarstein LJ, eds. New York, Masson Publishing, pp 73-80.
26. Letvin NL, Eaton KA, Aldrich WR, et al. 1983. Acquired immunodeficiency syndrome in a colony of macaque monkeys. Proc Natl Acad Sci USA 80:2718-2722.
27. Giddens WE, Morton WR, Hefti E, Panem S, Ochs H. 1983. Enzootic retroperitoneal fibromatosis in *Macaca* spp. In: Viral and Immunological Diseases in Nonhuman Primates. New York, Alan R Liss Inc, pp 249-253.
28. Henrickson R, Maul DH, Osborn KG, et al. 1983. Epidemic of acquired immunodeficiency in rhesus monkeys. Lancet 1:388-390.
29. Marx PA, Maul DH, Osborn KG, Lerche NW, Moody P, Lowenstein LJ, Henrickson RV. 1984. Simian AIDS: Isolation of a type D retrovirus and disease transmission. Science 273:1084-1085.
30. London WT, Sever JL, Madden DL, et al. 1983. Experimental transmission of simian acquired immune deficiency syndrome (SAIDS) and Kaposi-like skin lesions. Lancet 2:869-873.
31. Gravell M, London WR, Houff SA, et al. 1984. Transmission of simian acquired immunodeficiency syndrome (SAIDS) with blood or filtered plasma. Science 223:74-76.
32. Metroka CE, Cunningham-Rundles S, Pollack MS, Sonnabend JA,

Davis JM, Gordon B, Fernandez RD, Mouradian J. 1983. Generalized lymphadenopathy in homosexual men. Ann Intern Med 99:585-591.

33. Meyer PR, Ormerod D, Osborn KG, et al. 1985 (in press). An immunopathologic evaluation of lymph nodes from monkey and man with the acquired immune deficiency syndrome and related conditions. Hematol Oncol
34. Osborn KG, Meyer PR, Ormerod LD, et al. 1985 (submitted). Lymph node-based pathogenesis of simian acquired immune deficiency syndrome (SAIDS) in rhesus monkeys: a morphologic/immunohistochemical characterization with clinical, immune and viral correlation.
35. Pitchenik AE, Fischel MA, Spira TJ. 1983. Acquired immune deficiency syndrome in low-risk patients. J Am Med Assoc 250:1310-1312.
36. Levine AM, Meyer PR, Gill PS, Burkes RL, Krailo M, Aguilar S, Parker JW. 1985 (submitted). Importance of diagnostic lymph node biopsy in homosexual men with generalized lymphadenopathy.
37. Meyer PR, Yanagihara ET, Parker JW, Lukes RJ. 1984 (in press). A distinctive follicular hyperplasia in the acquired immune deficiency syndrome (AIDS) and the AIDS-related complex. Hematol Oncol
38. Davis JM, Mouradian J, Reinandez RD, Metroka C. 1984. Acquired immune deficiency syndrome. Arch Surg 119:90-95.
39. Modlin RL, Hofman FM, Meyer PR, et al. 1983. Altered distribution of B and T lymphocytes in lymph nodes from homosexual men with Kaposi's sarcoma. Lancet 2:768-771.
40. Ziegler JL, Beckstead JA, Volberding PA, et al. 1984. Non-Hodgkin's lymphoma in 90 homosexual men: relationship to generalized lymphadenopathy and the acquired immunodeficiency syndrome. N Eng J Med 311:565-570.
41. Burkes R, Levine AM, Meyer PR, et al. 1985 (in press). Development of B-cell lymphoma in two monogamous homosexual men. Arch Int Med (in press).
42. Levine AM, Gill PS, Meyer PR, et al. 1985 (in press). Human T-lymphotrophic virus (HTLV-III) associated malignant lymphoma in homosexual men.
43. Lerche NW, Osborn KG, Marx PA, Prahalada S, Maul DH, Lowenstine LJ, Hendrickson RV. 1985 (submitted). An inapparent carrier state in simian AIDS and evidence for natural transmission through saliva.
44. Groopman JE, Salahuddin SZ, Sarngadharan MG, Markham PD, Gonda M, Sliski A, Gallo RC. 1984. HTLV-III in saliva of people with AIDS-related complex and healthy homosexual men at risk for AIDS. Science 226:447-449.
45. Zagury D, Bernard J, Leibowitch J, Safai B, Groopman JE, Feldman M, Sarngadharan MG, Gallo RC. 1984. HTLV-III in cells cultured from semen of two patients with AIDS. Science 226:449-451.
46. Ho DD, Schooley RT, Rota TR, et al. 1984. HTLV-III in the semen and blood of a healthy homosexual man. Science 226:451-453.
47. Alter HJ, Eichberg JW, Masur H, Saxinger WC, Gallo R, Macher AM, Lane HC, Fauci AS. 1984. Transmission of HTLV-III infection from human plasma to chimpanzees: An animal model for AIDS. Science 226:549-552.

HUMAN T-LYMPHOTROPIC RETROVIRUS (HTLV-III) ASSOCIATED LYMPHOPROLIFERATIVE DISORDERS IN HOMOSEXUAL MEN

ALEXANDRA M. LEVINE, PARKASH GILL, PAUL MEYER, SURAIYA RASHEED

Acquired immunodeficiency syndrome (AIDS) has been defined, operationally by the Center for Disease Control (CDC), as the development of opportunistic infections and/or Kaposi's sarcoma in an individual who is not at risk for these disorders.[1] As of September, 1984, approximately 6,000 cases of AIDS had been reported in the United States.[2] Aside from the classic AIDS group, a far larger group of individuals currently exist, who do not meet the CDC criteria for AIDS, but who have various conditions which have been termed part of the AIDS-related complex (ARC). These conditions include other neoplasms, a syndrome of persistent, generalized lymphadenopathy (PGL), immune thrombocytopenic purpura, and other immune or auto-immune disorders. These disorders are currently not reportable to the CDC, and precise numbers of affected individuals are not known. It is presumed, however, that far greater numbers of patients currently have one of these ARC disorders as compared to the known AIDS group.

Persistent, generalized lymhadenopathy (PGL) has been defined by the CDC as the occurrence of lymphadenopathy involving two or more extra-inguinal sites, of at least three months duration, in the absence of any known intercurrent illness known to cause lymphadenopathy.[3] Morphologically, the involved lymph nodes were said to be benign and reactive. Subsequent to the initial definition of PGL, various investigators have described the specific morphologic abnormalities in PGL more carefully;[4,5,6] these lymph nodes exhibit a characteristic, exuberant follicular hyperplasia, with disorganization and disruption of the reactive follicles. An evolution from the hyperplastic pattern to one of lymphoid depletion has also been described[6] and has been associated with subsequent poor prognosis.

The incidence of PGL in the homosexual population is largely unknown, although our experience would suggest that the syndrome may be relatively common. Thus, in a recent evaluation of normal, healthy, asymptomatic homosexual men from Los Angeles County, 5/14 (36%) were found to have lymphadenopathy on physical examination.

We began a study of the natural history of PGL in homosexual men approximately one year ago. Thirty-four patients have now been entered on study and form the basis for the following information. All patients underwent initial lymph node biopsy to confirm the diagnosis of PGL. The epidemiologic profile of these patients was quite uniform. All were homosexual or bisexual males and all had a history of receptor anal intercourse. Anonymous, promiscuous sexual contact was practiced by all, with a mean number of lifetime male sexual partners of 682, and median of 200. All patients gave histories of illicit "recreational" drug abuse, including marijuana, cocaine, amyl nitrite, and amphetamine in the majority.

The initial symptoms included fever (47%), night sweats (35%), headache with photophobia (18%), and extreme malaise (53%). Significant weight loss was reported by 24% of these patients, while diarrhea was noted in 21%. The majority of patients first noted the onset of lymphadenopathy after the onset of fever, sweats and malaise. The lymph nodes were noted to be tender at the outset, and then became non-tender and non-painful to palpation. The majority of patients have described fluctuation of lymph node size in time, with recurrence of tenderness and increasing lymph node size associated with fatigue, stress, and increasing drug abuse. The mean duration of these symptoms prior to diagnostic lymph node biopsy was 7.6 months (range 0.65-37.9). The duration of symptoms and signs of disease is unknown at this time, but is at least one to two years, as evidenced by this group of patients.

On physical examination, the lymph nodes are large (two centimeters or more), firm, and rubbery. Axillary lymphadenopathy was present in 30, inguinal in 29, cervical in 29, submandibular in six, occipital in seven, epitrochlear in three (9%), and supraclavicular in two (6%). Thus, unusual sites of reactive adenopathy, such as epitrochlear and supraclavicular areas, may be involved in PGL. Splenomegaly may also be seen in this disease, occurring in two patients (6%), while two patients were also noted to have hepatomegaly .

Immunologic studies on these patients have been of interest. The mean peripheral blood lymphocyte count was 2331/dl, with mean

T4 "helper" cells of 618/dl, mean T8 "suppressor" cells of 1128/dl, and mean T4/T8 ratio of 0.57 (range 0.2-1.2; normal 0.9-2.9). The majority of patients were found to have polyclonal hypergammaglobulinemia, with a mean gamma fraction in the peripheral blood of 2.1 gm/dl (normal of 0.7-1.7). The mean quantitative IgG was 2136 mg/dl (normal 600-2000), with a mean IgA of 236 mg/dl (normal 50-400), and mean IgM of 147 mg/dl (normal 40-250). All precipitin arcs were normal in configuration. In vitro study of lymphocyte function revealed significantly increased spontaneous IgG synthesis (>1000 ng/2X10^5 PBM) by B-lymphocytes in eight of 13 PGL patients, and, paradoxically, all but two had decreased pokeweed mitogen (PWM)-induced IgG synthesis. Mean interleukin-1 production was significantly lower in PGL (57% of normal) when compared to 16 patients with AIDS (71% of normal; $p<.05$). In contrast, interleukin-2 levels were significantly lower in AIDS when compared to PGL (30% versus 218%; $p<.05$).

All patients had evidence of prior infection with Epstein-Barr virus (EBV), with serologic patterns consistent with reactivation or immune compromise in two of these. Likewise, the vast majority of patients had been exposed to the human T-lymphotropic retrovirus (HTLV-III), with antibody against sucrose-density banded, whole, purified virus detected by the enzyme-linked immunosorbent assay (ELISA) method in 95%. Interestingly, this antibody may not confer protection against the virus, as live virus has been grown from blood and saliva in two of our patients, who have had the highest antibody levels, documented since 1982, with live virus detected in 1984.

The eventual outcome of patients with PGL is largely unknown at this time, as is the relationship between PGL and AIDS. In 42 patients reported by Mathur-Wagh et al,[7] eight patients (19%) subsequently evolved from PGL to AIDS. It should be noted that only 26/42 patients actually underwent initial diagnostic lymph node biopsy. Of 90 PGL patients reported by Metroka et al,[8] 15 (17%) evolved to AIDS. Seventy-seven of these patients underwent initial lymph node biopsy. In 70 patients reported by Abrams et al,[9] evolution from PGL to AIDS was documented in none. Again, only half of the PGL study population (35) actually underwent initial diagnostic lymph node biopsy. The importance of initial node biopsy in homosexual men with lymphadenopathy may be illustrated by our current study. Thus, of the first 40 patients evaluated as potential PGL study participants, six were excluded from study when results of lymph node biopsy revealed lesions other than PGL. Malignant lymphoma was found on biopsy in two of these patients, Kaposi's sarcoma in two, disseminated tuberculosis in one, and disseminated histoplasmosis in one. No pre-biopsy clinical or laboratory parameter could predict the finding of PGL versus one of these other diagnoses. When one considers the question of evolution from PGL to AIDS, then it becomes critical to have documented that the patients in question did, in fact, have PGL at the outset. If initial biopsy had not been performed on all 40 of our potential study patients, for example, the eventual diagnosis of AIDS would have been made in six (15%); in fact, AIDS was present at the outset in these patients. With average follow-up periods ranging from one to two years, then, the vast majority of PGL patients do not appear to experience evolution to AIDS. The potential evolution of these individuals from PGL to malignant lymphoma is another issue of interest. When one considers the fact that these patients are immuno-compromised, with spontaneous hyperactivity of the B-lymphoid system, the potential for malignant transformation is apparent. In fact, the development of malignant lymphoma has already occurred in one of our PGL study patients. This individual was initially evaluated in March, 1984. His lymph node biopsy was consistent with PGL, revealing exuberant follicular hyperplasia. Peripheral blood lymphocyte count was 1221/dl, with a T4"helper":-T8"suppressor" ratio of 0.3. Significant polyclonal hypergammaglobulinemia was present, with a quantitative IgG level of 6830 mg/dl. Serologic analysis for Epstein-Barr virus was consistent with reactivation, with anti-EB viral capsid antigen (VCA) of 1:10,240, and antibody of the restricted portion of the early EBV antigen of 1:40. Antibody to HTLV-III was present in high titer. In July of 1984, a repeat lymph node biopsy had changed to reveal a pattern of lymphoid depletion. The quantitative IgG had risen to 8190 mg/dl, and the T4:T8 ratio had fallen to <0.1. An abdominal mass was detected in August, 1984. Diagnostic laparotomy revealed a B-cell immunoblastic sarcoma from which the patient expired in October, 1984, in spite of multi-agent chemotherapy.

Indeed, the occurrence of non-Hodgkin's lymphoma in patients at risk for AIDS has raised the possibility that lymphoma may, in fact, be one facet of the current AIDS epidemic. The initial report of non-Hodgkin's lymphoma in homosexual men was published by Ziegler et al in 1982, who noted the occurrence of undifferentiated Burkitt-like lymphomas in four homosexual men.[10] Levine et al subsequently described aggressive, extranodal lymphomas of B-lymphoid origin in six such patients,[11] and a further collaborative study described the development of malignant lymphoma in 90 homosexual men in San Francisco, Los Angeles, Houston, and New York.[12] Recent data from the University of Southern California Cancer Surveillance Program, the population based cancer registry for Los Angeles County, has indicated an increased incidence of B-cell immunoblastic sarcoma and small non-cleaved lymphoma (either Burkitt or Burkitt-like) since 1981 in never-married males,[13] and similar information has also been reported from San Francisco.[12] It is likely, then, that the spectrum of AIDS does include malignant lymphoma. Problematically, however, it does not seem appropriate to designate any homosexual man with lymphoma as having AIDS, and the precise characteristics of AIDS-related lymphomas must be defined.

Over the past two years, we have cared for 27 homosexual men with malignant lymphoma, whose initial diagnosis was made in our Institution. From a careful evaluation of the clinical, pathologic, immunologic and virologic details of disease in these patients, we have been able to elucidate those factors which serve to define the AIDS-related lymphomas. These factors will herein be discussed.

Prior to the diagnosis of lymphoma, seven patients had histories of opportunistic infection and/or Kaposi's sarcoma, which would have allowed a diagnosis of AIDS. Two additional patients were diagnosed simultaneously with Kaposi's sarcoma and lymphoma, while a third such patient was diagnosed simultaneously with lymphoma, Kaposi's sarcoma, cytomegalovirus infection, and pneumocystis carinii pneumonia. Thus, a total of 10/27 (37%) had prior or simultaneous evidence of AIDS.

The mean age of these 27 patients was 37 years (range 21-61). There were 19 Caucasians, two Blacks, and six Hispanics. Systemic "B" symptoms were common, present at diagnosis in 20 (74%). These consisted of fever in 16 (59%), weight loss in 11 (41%), night sweats in nine (33%). Fourteen patients complained of significant fatigue at presentation.

The epidemiologic factors present in these patients were quite similar to what has previously been described in AIDS. All patients were homosexual or bisexual, and all engaged in anonymous sexual contact. The mean number of different like-time sexual partners was 172, with a median of 80. All patients had a history of receptive anal intercourse. All but one patient admitted to the use of various "recreational" street drugs. Two patients used intravenous heroin.

The pathologic evaluation of these patients was quite interesting. The diagnosis of B-cell immunoblastic sarcoma (B-IBS) was made in 11 patients (41%), while small non-cleaved follicular center cell lymphoma (SNC) was found in 11 (41%). Indolent or low grade types of lymphoma were diagnosed in the remaining five individuals in the series (19%), including three cases with small cleaved follicular center cell lymphoma (SC-FCC), and two with plasmacytoid-lymphocytic (P-L) lymphoma. One patient with small cleaved lymphoma was initially untreated, and experienced transformation to a high-grade small non-cleaved, non-Burkitt tumor, ten months after initial presentation. The distribution of pathologic types of disease is most unusual, when compared to prior series of non-Hodgkin's lymphoma. In a previous series of 425 cases of lymphoma from this institution, the incidence of B-IBS was 3.5%, while small non-cleaved (SNC) lymphoma comprised 6.8% of the total group.[14] The National Cancer Institute (NCI)-sponsored study of 1175 lymphoma cases from four institutions revealed small non-cleaved lymphoma in 5% of all cases, and immunoblastic lymphoma (including both T-cell and B-cell disease) in 7.9%.[15] The small cleaved cell type was most commonly encountered, diagnosed in 29.4% of the NCI series, and in 28% of the series reported by Lukes et al.[14,15] By contrast, this usual distribution of pathologic types is not apparent in the current series. Thus, the high-grade types (B-IBS and SNC) accounted for 82% of the cases, while the small cleaved variant was found in only three patients, or 11%. The unusual pathologic spectrum of disease is a distinguishing feature of the AIDS-related lymphomas.

On morphologic grounds, all lymphomas in the current series were of B-lymphoid type. Immunoglobulin phenotype studies were performed on 24 cases, and the B-cell nature of disease was confirmed in 23. Nineteen of these cases were monoclonal by light chain staining.

At staging evaluation, extranodal disease was present in 23 patients (85%), while disease limited to lymph nodes was found in only four (15%). This distribution of stage is most unusual, when compared to prior series of non-Hodgkin's lymphoma. Thus, in a series of 405 patients with newly diagnosed lymphoma reported by Jones et al,[16] disease limited to lymph nodes alone (Stage I, II, III) was found in 61%, while only six patients (1%) were found to have localized extranodal disease (IE) at initial presentation. In contrast, only 15% of the patients in the current series presented with lymphoma confined to nodal sites. In our 27 patients, stage IV was present in 17 (63%), consisting of involvement of the bone marrow in six, gastrointestinal tract in six (small bowel in four, rectum and skin in one, rectum and bowel in one), and miscellaneous sites in five. Three of these patients also had initial involvement of the central nervous system (CNS). The remaining six patients presented with stage IE disease, involving CNS alone in five, and isolated involvement of the anus in one. Again, involvement of these unusual sites of extranodal disease serves to distinguish the current patients from what is ordinarily expected in non-Hodgkin's lymphoma. Thus, in a prior report from this institution, malignant lymphoma primary to the rectum or anus was described in eight patients, whose diagnosis was made over a ten-year period of time.[17] In the current series, we report three cases diagnosed within one year. Central nervous system, as well, is an unusual site of initial lymphomatous presentation, reported at diagnosis in 8.6% of diffuse histiocytic cases, and in 12% of diffuse undifferentiated lymphoma.[18] In the current series, initial CNS involvement was detected in eight patients, or 30%. Occurrence of lymphoma in unusual extranodal sites, such as CNS and rectum, then, is one distinguishing clinical feature of the AIDS-related lymphomas.

The majority of our patients were not normal immunologically at initial presentation. The mean absolute lymphocyte count in the peripheral blood was 1335/dl (range 84-4284). The mean absolute T4 "helper" cells was 352/dl (range 16-1927), with a mean absolute T8 "suppressor" cell count of 733/dl (range 43-2270). The mean ratio of T4:T8 cells was 0.5 (range 0.03-2.2:Normal=0.9-2.9). Only three patients had normal T4:T8 ratios.

Serum protein electrophoresis, and quantitative immunoglobulins were performed on 17 patients. The mean gamma fraction was 2.02 gm/dl (range 0.9-7.4:Normal=0.7-1.7). The mean quantitative IgG was 2045 mg/dl (range 687-7710:Normal=600-2000). Mean IgA was 249 mg/dl (range 60-651:Normal=50-400). Mean IgM was 156 mg/dl (range 77-401:Normal=40-250). All precipitin arcs were normal in configuration.

Since HTLV-III has been reported as a possible etiologic agent of AIDS and related disorders,[19] we tested the patient and various control sera for the presence of antibodies to this virus. Serum from 20 patients was tested, and revealed the presence of antibody against HTLV-III in 15 (75%). Of 15 patients with high-grade lymphoma tested (B-IBS or SNC), 13 had antibody to HTLV-III (87%), compared to 2/5 (40%) patients with low-grade disease. Moreover, one of the low-grade cases had simultaneous onset of Kaposi's sarcoma and lymphoma, which would have allowed a diagnosis of AIDS. In 40 heterosexual, asymptomatic health care workers tested, none was positive (p<.001). Of seven heterosexual patients, with no known risk factor for AIDS, diagnosed with B-IBS or SNC lymphoma in our institution in 1984, none was positive for antibodies to HTLV-III (P<.001). In seven heterosexual patients with no known risk factor for AIDS, diagnosed with B-IBS or SNC lymphoma in the late 1970's, one was positive (14%;P=.002). The difference between these control groups and the current patients is highly significant.

Serum antibodies against the Epstein-Barr virus were tested in 18 patients. All patients tested had sustained prior EBV infection, and the majority had antibody patterns and titers within the range of healthy sero-positive individuals. Only five patients showed evidence of possible reactivation, with increase in either EB-viral capsid antigen (VCA), anti-restricted portion of the early antigen (anti-R) or both. Touch preparations from lymphomatous tissue of six patients were tested for the presence of EBV nuclear antigen, and were negative in all.

Serum from 22 patients was tested for the presence of antibody or antigen to the hepatitis B virus. Twenty-one (95%) had been infected at some time with hepatitis B virus. Seven of these patients (33%) were positive for hepatitis B surface antigen, but were anicteric and had liver enzyme studies consistent with chronic hepatitis B infection, indicating possible chronic carrier state or underlying immunosuppression. The role of hepatitis B virus as sole etiologic agent in these lymphomas would thus be unlikely.

Antibody analysis for cytomegalovirus (CMV) was performed in 18 patients, and was consistent with prior infection in 16, with elevation of IgG, but not IgM anti-CMV antibody. Acute CMV infection was present in two of the current patients; both of these patients had prior or simultaneous diagnosis of AIDS. Since CMV infection was not present acutely in the majority of patients, this organism would most likely not be the sole etiologic factor in the development of lymphoma in our patients.

Two patients in the series had the diagnosis of lymphoma made only at autopsy, and two patients expired within one week of presentation. Four additional patients, with low-grade lymphoma and asymptomatic disease, were left untreated. Thus, 19 patients received treatment for lymphoma. The M-BACOD regimen[20] was administered to nine patients. Three of these remain on therapy. Three patients attained complete remission; one has subsequently relapsed and the others remain without disease 12+ and 18+ months from diagnosis. Three patients had disease progression while on M-BACOD, occurring in CNS, bone marrow and peripheral nodes, respectively.

Seven patients received either CHOP[21] or BACOP,[22] resulting in complete remission in two. One has relapsed in the CNS, and the second remains tumor free 11 months after end of therapy. One patient attained partial remission, and the remaining four experienced no response, with disease progression in the central nervous system in two of the latter cases.

The COM regimen[23] was used in one patient, who presented with small non-cleaved lymphoma in the leukemia phase; the regimen was ineffective. Two patients with primary CNS lymphoma were treated with cranial radiation: one experienced no response, and the second, with indolent pathologic disease (P-L), attained complete remission and remains disease free 28+ months from the end of treatment.

Thus, disease progression or relapse isolated to the CNS occurred in four of the treated patients, including one patient who received high dose methotrexate as part of his systemic chemotherapy. A total of 12 patients in the series (44%) experienced disease in the central nervous system at some time during the course of disease, making early treatment of this site mandatory.

With a median follow-up of eight months, 13 patients in the series have died (48%), 10 due to lymphoma. Three patients in the current report have died of infection; none of these had received treatment for lymphoma, each having presented simultaneously with lymphoma and opportunistic infections consistent with AIDS. It is important to recognize that these patients have not died of granulocytopenia and sepsis secondary to chemotherapy, but rather, of malignant lymphoma, in spite of aggressive, multi-agent chemotherapy. Results of newer therapeutic modalities are awaited with interest. The median survival for all patients in the series is eight months.

It is thus apparent that the AIDS-related malignant lymphomas occurring in homosexual men are unique, both pathologically and clinically, when compared to prior series of non-Hodgkin's lymphoma. These patients present with high-grade lymphomas, in unusual extranodal sites, such as CNS and/or rectum, reversed T "helper":T "suppressor" ratios in the blood, and exposure to HTLV-III. Further, these specific characteristics may serve to define the individual cases which are related to the current AIDS epidemic.

The association of HTLV-III and development of malignant lymphoma in these patients is of interest in an etiologic sense. Of 20 patients tested, only five lacked antibody to this virus. Interestingly, three of these antibody-negative patients were the only individuals in the study who had normal T "helper":T "suppressor" ratios in the peripheral blood. Further, two of these had indolent lymphomas, and the third was one of only four patients in the series who presented with disease confined to lymph nodes. It is very possible that these individuals, although homosexual, did not have disease which would be considered part of the current AIDS-related epidemic. One additional patient lacked antibody against HTLV-III. This patient was tested after failing four months of multi-agent chemotherapy; he may have been unable to mount an antibody response. In contrast, of five current patients with indolent lymphomas, only two had antibody to HTLV-III

(40%;p=.07). Further, striking differences are apparent in the prevalence of antibody to HTLV-III among the current patients with high-grade lymphoma and other patients with identical types of lymphoma, who were heterosexual, and in whom no risk factor was apparent for the development of AIDS. Thus, the high-grade lymphomas developing in homosexual men are clearly associated with exposure to HTLV-III, an agent which may, in fact, be causative. The potential etiologic relationship between HTLV-III and malignant lymphoma in out-patients is further strengthened by the recent evidence that simian AIDS (SAIDS) is caused by a related retrovirus,[24] which, if injected into normal monkeys, may cause malignant lymphoma of the same high-grade pathologic types as described in the current series of patients.[25]

The lymphomas in the current series were of B-lymphoid origin, which is most interesting when one considers that HTLV-III is a T-cell trophic virus, specifically capable of infecting T4-positive helper cells.[26] In this regard, the recent report by Montagnier et al[27] is of relevance. These investigators found that the lymphadenopathy virus (LAV), which is closely related and possibly identical to HTLA-III, can infect EBV-infected B-lymphoblastoid cell lines. These EBV-infected B-cell lines become particularly potent producers of LAV. In the current series, all patients tested had evidence of prior EBV infection. However, EBNA staining of involved tissue was negative in all six cases studied, although four of these were of indolent pathologic type. It would thus appear that Epstein-Barr virus is an unlikely candidate as sole etiologic agent. It is known that EBV is capable of infecting and immortalizing B lymphocytes. Perhaps the B-cell proliferation induced by EBV, associated with the immunosuppressive effects of HTLV-III and the lifestyle habits of these patients, could provide the appropriate setting in which malignant transformation of HTLV-III-infected B lymphocytes could occur. Further tests will be needed to evaluate these and other possibilities.

REFERENCES

1. Follow-up on Kaposi's sarcoma and Pneumocystis pneumonia. 1981. MMWR 30:409-410.
2. Monthly report. 1984. Public Health Department, Los Angeles County, California.

3. Persistent, generalized lymphadenopathy among homosexual males. 1982. MMWR 31:249-251.
4. Meyer PR, Yanagihara E, Taylor CR, Parker JW, Lukes RJ. Abnormal B-cell proliferation in AIDS and related disorders with evolution of B cell lymphoma: An immunomorphologic study of lymph node biopsies in 29 cases. In press. Hematol Oncol.
5. Brynes RK, Chan WC, Spira TJ, et al. 1983. Value of lymph node biopsy in unexplained lymphadenopathy in homosexual men. J Amer Med Assoc 250:1313-1317.
6. Fernandez R, Mouradian J, Metroka C, Davis J. 1983. The prognostic value of histopathology in persistent generalized lymphadenopathy in homosexual males. (Letter) N Engl J Med 309:185-186.
7. Mathur-Wagh U, Spigland I, Sacks HS, et al. 1984. Longitudinal study of persistent, generalized lymphadenopathy in homosexual men: Relation to acquired immunodeficiency syndrome. Lancet 2:1033-1038.
8. Metroka CE, Cunningham-Rundles S, Pollack MS, et al. 1983. Generalized lymphadenopathy in homosexual men. Ann Intern Med 99:585-591.
9. Abrams DI, Lewis BJ, Beckstead JH, Casavant CA, Drew WL. 1984. Persistent diffuse lymphadenopathy in homosexual men: Endpoint or prodrome? Ann Intern Med 100:801-808.
10. Ziegler JL, Drew WL, Miner RC, et al. 1982. Outbreak of Burkitt's-like lymphoma in homosexual men. Lancet 2:631-633.
11. Levine AM, Meyer PR, Begandy MK, et al. 1984. Development of B-cell lymphoma in homosexual men: Clinical and immunologic findings. Ann Intern Med 100:7-13.
12. Ziegler JL, Beckstead JA, Volberding PA, et al. 1984. Non-Hodgkin's lymphoma in 90 homosexual men: Relationship to generalized lymphadenopathy and acquired immunodeficiency syndrome. N Engl J Med 311:565-570.
13. Ross R. Cancer Surveillance Registry, Los Angeles County. Personal communication.
14. Lukes RJ, Parker JW, Taylor CR, Tindle BH, Cramer AD, Lincoln TD. 1978. Immunologic approach to non-Hodgkin's lymphomas and related leukemias. Analysis of the results of multiparameter studies of 425 cases. Semin Hematol 15:322-351.
15. Non-Hodgkin's lymphoma pathologic classification project: National Cancer Institute sponsored study of classifications of non-Hodgkin's lymphomas: Summary and description of a Working Formulation for Clinical Usage. 1982. Cancer 49:2112-2135.
16. Jones SE, Fuks Z, Bull M, et al. 1973. Clinicopathologic correlation in 405 cases. Cancer 31:806-823.
17. Vanden Huele B, Taylor CR, Terry R, Lukes RJ. 1982. Presentation of malignant lymphoma in the rectum. Cancer 49:2602-2607.
18. Mackintosh, FR, Colby TV, Podolsky WJ, et al. 1982. Central nervous system involvement in non-Hodgkin's lymphoma: An analysis of 105 cases. Cancer 49:586-595.
19. Popovic M, Sarngadharan MG, Read E, Gallo RC. 1984. Detection, isolation and continuous production of cytopathic retroviruses (HTLV-III) from patients with AIDS and pre-AIDS. Science 224:497-500.
20. Skarin AT, Canellos GP, Rosenthal DS, et al. 1983. Improved prognosis of diffuse histiocytic and undifferentiated lymphoma by use of high dose methotrexate alternating with standard agents (M-BACOD). J Clin Oncol 1:91-98.
21. McKelvey EM, Gottlieb JA, Wilson HE, et al. 1976. Hydroxyldaunomycin (adriamycin) combination chemotherapy in malignant

lymphoma. Cancer 38:1484-1493.
22. Schein PS, DeVita VT Jr, Hubbard S, et al. 1976. Bleomycin, adriamycin, cyclophosphamide, vincristine, and prednisone (BACOP) combination chemotherapy in the treatment of advanced diffuse histiocytic lymphoma. Ann Intern Med 85:417-422.
23. Ziegler JL. 1977. Treatment results of 54 American patients with Burkitt's lymphoma are similar to the African experience. N Engl J Med 297:75-80.
24. Levitin NL, King NW, Daniel MD, Aldrich WR, Blake BJ, Junt RD. 1983. Experimental transmission of macaque AIDS by means of innoculation of macaque lymphoma tissue. Lancet 2:599-602.
25. Hunt RD, Blake BJ, Chalifoux LV, Schgal PK, King NW, Levitin NL. 1983. Transmission of naturally occurring lymphoma in macaque monkeys. Proc Natl Acad Sci USA 80:5085-5089.
26. Barre-Sinoussi F, Chermann JC, Rey F, et al. 1983. Isolation of a T-lymphotropic retrovirus from a patient at risk for acquired immune deficiency syndrome (AIDS). Science 220:868-871.
27. Montagnier L, Gruest J, Chamaret S, et al. 1984. Adaptation of lymphadenopathy associated virus (LAV) to replication in EBV-transformed B-lymphoblastoid cell lines. Science 225:63-66.

Index of Subjects

GPSR Compliance

The European Union's (EU) General Product Safety Regulation (GPSR) is a set of rules that requires consumer products to be safe and our obligations to ensure this.

If you have any concerns about our products, you can contact us on ProductSafety@springernature.com

In case Publisher is established outside the EU, the EU authorized representative is:

Springer Nature Customer Service Center GmbH
Europaplatz 3
69115 Heidelberg, Germany

Batch number: 10761599

Printed by Printforce, the Netherlands